Humanitarian Programmes
and HIV and AIDS:
A Practical Approach to Mainstreaming

Oxfam GB

Oxfam GB, founded in 1942, is a development, humanitarian, and campaigning agency dedicated to finding lasting solutions to poverty and suffering around the world. Oxfam believes that every human being is entitled to a life of dignity and opportunity, and it works with others worldwide to make this become a reality.

From its base in Oxford in the United Kingdom, Oxfam GB publishes and distributes a wide range of books and other resource materials for development and relief workers, researchers and campaigners, schools and colleges, and the general public, as part of its programme of advocacy, education, and communications.

Oxfam GB is a member of Oxfam International, a confederation of 13 agencies of diverse cultures and languages, which share a commitment to working for an end to injustice and poverty – both in long-term development work and at times of crisis.

For further information about Oxfam's publishing, and online ordering, visit www.oxfam.org.uk/publications

For information about Oxfam's development, advocacy, and humanitarian relief work around the world, visit www.oxfam.org.uk

Humanitarian Programmes and HIV and AIDS: A Practical Approach to Mainstreaming

Vivien Margaret Walden, Marion O'Reilly, and Mary Yetter

Oxfam

First published by Oxfam GB in 2007

© Oxfam GB 2007

ISBN 978-0-85598-562-2

A catalogue record for this publication is available from the British Library.

Available from:

Bournemouth English Book Centre, PO Box 1496, Parkstone, Dorset, BH12 3YD, UK
tel: +44 (0)1202 712933; fax: +44 (0)1202 712930; email: oxfam@bebc.co.uk

USA: Stylus Publishing LLC, PO Box 605, Herndon, VA 20172-0605, USA
tel: +1 (0)703 661 1581; fax: +1 (0)703 661 1547; email: styluspub@aol.com

For details of local agents and representatives in other countries, consult our website:
www.oxfam.org.uk/publications
or contact Oxfam Publishing, Oxfam House, John Smith Drive, Cowley, Oxford,
OX4 2JY, UK
tel +44 (0) 1865 473727; fax (0) 1865 472393; email: publish@oxfam.org.uk

Our website contains a fully searchable database of all our titles, and facilities for secure on-line ordering.

Published by Oxfam GB, Oxfam House, John Smith Drive, Cowley, Oxford, OX4 2JY, UK

Printed by Information Press, Eynsham

Oxfam GB is a registered charity, no. 202 918, and is a member of Oxfam International.

Front cover: Volunteers help in the construction of a water tank, Kounoungo, Chad.
Carmen Rodrigues/Intermón Oxfam
Back cover: Nursing student, Malawi.
Eva-Lotta Jansson/Oxfam

Contents

List of acronyms

AIDS	acquired immunodeficiency syndrome
ART	antiretroviral therapy
ARV	antiretroviral drugs
CBO	community-based organisation
HIV	human immunodeficiency virus
IDP	internally displaced person
MMR	maternal mortality rate
MSM	men who have sex with men
MTCT	mother-to-child transmission
OCHA	United Nations Office for the Coordination of Humanitarian Affairs
OVC	orphans and other vulnerable children
PEP	post exposure prophylaxis
PLWHA	people living with HIV and AIDS
SGBV	sexual and gender-based violence
STI	sexually transmitted infection
TBA	traditional birth attendant
UNDP	United Nations Development Programme
VCT	voluntary counselling and testing
WHO	World Health Organization

Glossary of terms

asymptomatic
: The person is HIV-positive but is healthy and has not yet suffered from any of the conditions that are associated with AIDS.

commercial sex worker
: A person (male or female) who makes a living from paid sex.

food security
: Having access to enough food to stay healthy and active.

gender analysis
: Looks at the impact of HIV and AIDS on women and men in relation to their roles and status in society. Analyses how social and power relations between men and women are reflected in the differences in their vulnerability to infection, and the relevance of HIV and AIDS interventions to their needs and roles in the household, communities, and at the macro level.

HIV mainstreaming
: The process through which institutional capacity to cope with and respond to HIV is increased. It starts from existing work, which is then modified to take into account susceptibility and vulnerability to HIV and AIDS.

HIV profile
: The HIV and AIDS statistics for a particular country.

incidence
: The number of times an event occurs in a given time, e.g. the number of new AIDS cases presenting each month or year, or the number of new HIV infections being detected during a specified period of time.

opportunistic infections
: Parasitic, bacterial, viral, and fungal infections that can occur when the immune system is weakened. These infections may be resistant to treatment and may re-occur frequently.

prevalence
: The total number of specific HIV or AIDS conditions in existence in a defined population at a precise point in time, e.g. the number of AIDS cases or number of HIV infections which have so far been reported in a country. The systematic collection of facts (data) about disease occurrence is part of surveillance.

public health
: Promotion of health and prevention of disease through the organised efforts of society.

public health promotion
: (Oxfam term for health promotion.) The planned and systematic attempt to enable people to take action to prevent or mitigate disease.

sex for subsistence
: The trading of sexual favours for goods or services by people who do not consider themselves commercial sex workers.

syndrome
: A combination of signs and/or symptoms that forms a distinct clinical picture indicative of a particular disorder.

sentinel surveillance
: Periodic anonymous testing of a group of people in pre-selected sites to determine HIV prevalence in a country.

window period
: The period between infection with HIV and the detectable presence of antibodies to HIV. It lasts from several weeks to several months, during which the person is very infectious. The window period often includes an episode of illness resembling influenza.

Introduction

'My manager tells me to mainstream HIV and AIDS – how do I do it?' is a sentiment that echoes through many an emergency programme. No access to the Internet and a proposal to write – where do field staff turn for help?

Mainstreaming HIV and AIDS into humanitarian emergencies has been a challenge for many organisations and has not always been seen as an integral part of humanitarian response. Oxfam GB has made HIV and AIDS a cross-cutting organisational priority and has spent the past few years looking at ways of mainstreaming HIV and AIDS into all phases of a humanitarian response. This guide uses real examples from Oxfam programmes as well as fictitious examples based upon Oxfam's work in public health promotion, water and sanitation, and livelihoods. These examples include the broader picture of protection and gender in humanitarian settings.

This manual is aimed at humanitarian – and pre-dominantly rapid-onset – programmes in all countries. It is not intended to be used in chronic situations like the food crisis in Southern Africa where the level of HIV and AIDS prevalence warrants more focused programming. Nor is it intended to give guidance on implementing more targeted HIV and AIDS programming such as home-based care. However, should a rapid-onset emergency such as flooding occur in regions like Southern Africa, many of the principles of main-streaming would apply.

The manual is in six sections. Section 1 identifies the manual's target audience and describes what is meant by mainstreaming in emergencies. Section 2 explains both how HIV affects emergencies and how emergencies affect HIV, as well as potential vulnerable groups. Section 3 describes mainstreaming throughout the project cycle as well as specific sectoral responses. Section 4 is intended to guide managers in their planning. Section 5 is a resource section with examples of inductions, trainings, and awareness-raising sessions both for staff and for community members. Appendix 4 includes cards which can be photocopied and used for these activities. Section 6 is a short summary of important points. There is also a glossary and list of acronyms in the front of the manual.

The manual does not include statistics or clinical information – sources for these can be found elsewhere (for example on the UNAIDS and WHO websites) and references are included in the bibliography. There is a short appendix on facts about HIV and AIDS.

The authors wish to thank the following people for their input or comments: Miriam Aschkenasy (Oxfam America), Nega Bazazew, Jane Beesley, Sally Crook, Mary Davies, Judith Flick, Cathy Gibb, Rachel Hastie, Lucy Heaven, Jesse Kinyanjui Wainaina, Martin Knops, Chris Leather, Olwyn Mason, Auriol Miller, Wayne Myslik, Maren Lieberum, Silke Pietzsch, Laura Phelps, Jo Podlesak, Christina Schmalenbach, Ines Smythe, Foyeke Tolani, Marilise Turnbull, and all the participants at the Regional Humanitarian Co-ordinator meeting in Nairobi. We would also like to acknowledge the work of Kathleen Skinner who wrote the first HIV and AIDS mainstreaming manual for Oxfam.

Special thanks go to Kondwani Mwangulube from the International HIV/AIDS Alliance for his invaluable input and to Fiona Perry from Tearfund for her comments.

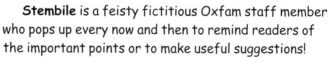

Stembile is a feisty fictitious Oxfam staff member who pops up every now and then to remind readers of the important points or to make useful suggestions!

Thanks to Pamela O'Honde for being the model for Stembile.

Section 1:
What is HIV and AIDS mainstreaming?

1.1 Who is this book for?

It is important that all emergency field staff including engineers, health promoters, managers, and co-ordinators have sufficient knowledge of HIV and AIDS in order to plan and implement a mainstreamed humanitarian programme. This manual is primarily based on Oxfam experiences, and the learning and examples of good practice will be useful for all organisations who have field staff working in humanitarian programmes.

Emergency programmes in areas such as Haiti and Cambodia, where there is a high prevalence of HIV, will have different needs from those in a low-prevalence country such as Guatemala. This means that field staff will of course have to use their discretion about when and how a programme mainstreams HIV and AIDS. Section 3.2 (page 21) contains clear guidelines on how to make an informed choice.

1.2 What is mainstreaming?

Mainstreaming has been defined as 'The application of learning and new behaviours into core activities of organisations.'[1] For example, gender can be mainstreamed into humanitarian programmes by promoting equality for both sexes throughout the life of the programme rather than attempting to run parallel projects for empowering women. Protection issues such as the safety of women and the prevention of rape are mainstreamed into programmes by reshaping the interventions to minimise risks and to increase safety: an example being well-lit sanitation facilities for women and children in refugee camps. So the objective to address the immediate needs of the affected people remains, but the programme is designed to address gender and protection at all stages.

In order to be able to mainstream HIV and AIDS, we need to be clear about two different definitions: **HIV and AIDS programming** and **mainstreaming HIV and AIDS**. Holden (2004) has come up with the following differences:

1   The term **HIV and AIDS programming** refers to HIV prevention and treatment, care and support for people living with HIV and AIDS (PLWHA), or HIV and AIDS-focused interventions that are integrated within broader health and related programming. The goal of HIV and AIDS programming relates specifically to HIV and AIDS.

2   The term **mainstreaming HIV and AIDS** refers to 'adapting development and humanitarian programmes to ensure they address the underlying causes of vulnerability to HIV infection and the consequences of HIV/AIDS' (Holden 2004: 40). The focus of such programmes, however, remains the original goal (in the case of Oxfam providing water, sanitation, and hygiene promotion as well as livelihoods, for example).

Stembile says:

It's like putting on HIV glasses and viewing your programme from a different angle!

The Sphere Project is used in humanitarian programmes as a gold standard for good programming and it includes HIV and AIDS mainstreaming. According to Sphere, 'action must be taken in the acute stage following the disaster to minimise risk of (HIV) infection' and 'a basic response to any emergency must aim to maintain respect for the individual rights of people with HIV infection or AIDS'.[2]

Within an NGO emergency programme, HIV and AIDS mainstreaming is usually seen as both internal and external:

- **Internal** – addressing HIV and AIDS with staff through training on self-awareness and community mainstreaming, adapting and changing policy to promote staff welfare

- **External** – reducing the risk or the impact of HIV and AIDS through the way we interact with communities and deliver our programmes

1.3 HIV and emergencies

Box 1: Three Scenarios

1. **HIV and AIDS as an emergency** – for example the Southern Africa HIV and AIDS epidemic

2. **HIV and AIDS in an emergency** – for example the Sudan conflict where HIV rates are low but the conflict has the potential for increasing the rates

3. **HIV and AIDS as an emergency in an emergency** – for example the Southern Africa food crisis where pre-crisis HIV rates are high and the emergency will very probably increase the rates

This manual deals primarily with the second scenario – rapid-onset or protracted and complex emergencies.

Mainstreaming HIV in the second scenario (Box 1) is important because the emergency may increase transmission and thereby susceptibility to disease in people already affected by the crisis. In scenario three, the one emergency (HIV and AIDS crisis) will affect the other emergency (food shortage) and vice versa.

Other issues that must be considered when mainstreaming HIV are gender and protection.[3] Addressing these factors helps to decrease the chances of becoming infected and to mitigate the impacts of the virus. Managers often struggle with the problem of deciding **when to intervene** and **at what level**. A Scoring Tool has been developed to help make those decisions – see page 24.

Three primary principles of mainstreaming HIV and AIDS in emergencies are:

1 **Prevention of HIV transmission:** This can be achieved by promoting health and strengthening food security and livelihood security, with a focus on women and vulnerable groups. This will be important in decreasing behaviour that increases HIV transmission risks (e.g. sex for subsistence as a survival strategy and forced migration in search of employment). Safe blood transfusions will also prevent transmission and even those NGOs not involved in medical services should lobby for safe blood products.

2 **Care of both infected and affected:** A nutritionally balanced diet mitigates the health impact of AIDS (opportunistic infections[4]), so promoting health and good nutrition is important especially in an emergency. An issue that is often overlooked is support and assistance for carers of chronically ill people.[5] Addressing the special needs of chronically ill people by ensuring that water is easily available, for example, goes a long way in alleviating the burden of those who care for them.

3 **Mitigation of impact of the emergency on the HIV and AIDS profile:** This impact can be mitigated by alleviating labour loss and shortages, supporting livelihoods during the emergency-induced economic crisis, arresting agricultural disruption, and preventing sexual exploitation and rape (both male and female). Access to health services and antiretrovirals should also be considered, by humanitarian NGOs who have expertise in those areas.

1.4 What mainstreaming is not

- Working only with HIV-positive groups
- Running training courses on HIV prevention without using the knowledge to change the way we programme
- Doing mass condom distribution in isolation
- Changing the focus of the humanitarian response to HIV prevention

As Holden has stated: 'Mainstreaming is not concerned with completely changing an organisation's or sector's core functions and responsibilities, but with viewing them from a different perspective' (2004: 42). See Box 2 for an example of HIV mainstreaming.

Box 2: An example of HIV mainstreaming

In a cash-transfer programme, the vulnerable groups were defined as female-headed households, orphans and child-headed households, disabled and elderly as well as those selected by wealth ranking.

In an HIV-mainstreamed cash-transfer programme, the vulnerable groups also included those households with chronically ill people (those with a chronic illness that may or may not be due to AIDS).

Stembile says:

To sum it up – mainstreaming is thinking about HIV and AIDS in all programmes (and considering both staff and beneficiaries).

When considering any response you should ask yourself two key questions:

1) How will HIV and AIDS affect the programme?
2) How will the programme affect HIV and AIDS prevalence?

Section 2:
Why mainstream HIV and AIDS in emergencies?

2.1 Why get involved?

It is only in the past four or five years that it has become apparent that even in emergencies, programmes must consider HIV and AIDS. HIV and AIDS has not generally had a high profile in humanitarian programming. The reasons for this are:

- It is difficult to measure – due to poor surveillance and therefore poor data, few testing sites, and a mobile population.

- It is difficult to prevent transmission in a crisis – rape and sexual attack are more common, condoms may not be available, people use sex to barter for necessities, and prevention programmes are disrupted.

- It has been seen as a medical issue rather than a public health issue which affects sectors such as education, community, and livelihoods.

- It has been seen as a development and not an emergency issue; the increased risk of transmission linked to the presence of military, and an increase in rape cases have not often been considered in first-phase responses.

- It has not been seen as an immediately life-threatening disease such as malaria or cholera.

Nonetheless it is now recognised that HIV and AIDS can and must be mainstreamed into any emergency **analysis** and **response**. There is no point in saving lives in the short term if we fail to address the factors that may increase transmission (and thereby mortality rates) in emergencies. As one villager said during an assessment in Zimbabwe:

> 'We don't want to die with our bellies full.'

2.2 How emergencies can result in spreading HIV

Even before an emergency occurs, poverty, income inequality, gender inequity, poor public services, and low literacy all increase susceptibility to HIV infection, which in turn leads to a rise in opportunistic infections and death in the economically productive population (15–45 year olds). This then leads to decreased production; the cycle of poverty. Any emergency, whether due to natural disaster or conflict, will only worsen the situation.

Although conflict, poverty, food shortages, and displacement make people vulnerable, there is evidence to show that this vulnerability will not automatically result in increased HIV susceptibility. There have been cases when conflict has actually hindered the spread of HIV.[6] Figure 1 on page 11 illustrates how, in a conflict and/or displaced persons situation, while some factors may increase the risk of transmission, others will hinder the spread.

In all emergencies there is the potential for increased susceptibility to infection with HIV and increased vulnerability to the impacts of the HIV and AIDS epidemic. This is due to the following factors:

- Breakdown of family and social values and networks, with increased vulnerability and susceptibility especially of women and children
- Increase in rape cases often by military or paramilitary personnel[7]
- International military and sometimes international aid workers visiting local sex workers
- Breakdown in supply chain for condoms leading to more unprotected sex
- Poor IDP/refugee camp facilities, with latrines and washing areas for women unlit and far from the household, thus increasing the possibility of rape
- Breakdown in health services providing treatment for sexually transmitted infections (STIs) and other diseases

- No/limited access to antiretrovirals
- Tendency for men to seek work away from home in times of drought, leaving women and children to fend for themselves
- Tendency for migrant workers to visit commercial sex workers if they are forced to live far from their families
- Less disposable income, sometimes forcing women into sex for subsistence
- Coercion by aid workers distributing food or goods – workers asking for sexual favours or money in exchange for the food being distributed, or simply in exchange for registration for assistance[8]
- Increased blood transfusions due to large numbers of injured people in both conflict and natural disasters, in countries where there are poor blood screening facilities
- Interaction with host communities where transmission rates are higher than in the affected community[9]

Box 3 on page 12 gives examples of the impact of emergencies on HIV prevalence.

Figure 1: HIV risk factors in situations of conflict and displaced persons' camps

Key Factors

- HIV prevalence in area of origin (of displaced people)

- HIV prevalence in area of stay (host population/non-displaced population)

- Duration of emergency and therefore sustained vulnerability of affected community

Factors that can lead to an increase in risk

- Increased interaction between military and civilians

- Decreased availability of reproductive health and other services/means to prevent HIV transmission

- Decreased utilisation of reproductive health and other services/means to prevent HIV transmission

- Increased commercial and casual sex

- Increase in malnutrition

- Population movement/increased mixing of populations with different HIV prevalence

- Increased sexual violence, exploitation, rape as an instrument of war

Factors that can lead to a decrease in risk

- Isolation of communities

- High-risk groups may suffer increased death rates

- Decreased casual sex due to trauma and depression

- Improved protection and services in camps

- Disruption of sexual networks/partners

- Reduction in urbanization of communities

- Reduction in accessibility of populations (reduced trucking for example)

Source: P.B. Spiegel (2004) 'HIV/AIDS among conflict-affected and displaced populations: dispelling myths and taking action', *Disasters* 28 (3): 322–39.

Box 3: Impact of Emergencies on HIV Prevalence

Example of low impact

Aceh is a province in Indonesia that has been at war for 20 years. Despite the fact that reported HIV prevalence for the whole country is low, there is a lack of information around Aceh province. The war has meant that there is an influx of military personnel from other parts of the country including Java. There are reportedly high numbers of sex workers although this is difficult to confirm in a closed Muslim society where such activities are secret and socially unacceptable. Young men routinely leave the country for short periods – often illegally – to work in other countries such as Malaysia. During the tsunami in 2005, more women than men were killed, a fact that has resulted in hasty marriages between older widowers and young (sometimes orphaned) women. Two factors that could reduce transmission are the fact that Aceh is a 'dry state' (no alcohol[10]) and that the community is generally very close, with people looking after one another, so there is less risk of women resorting to sex for subsistence.

Example of medium impact

In Sierra Leone, displacement, the presence of foreign troops, increased sexual violence, lack of health services and a worsening economic situation have all fuelled the rise in HIV cases – although this is not as high as once feared.[11]

Example of high impact

In both Mozambique and Angola, prevalence rates were low during the conflict, but during post-conflict periods, the rates increased as refugees returned and movement within country was again possible.[12]

2.3 How HIV can aggravate the impact of emergencies

The effect of HIV on emergencies will depend on the prevalence in the country before the emergency. In a country with high prevalence there may already be a marked decrease in the number of young healthy workers in the agricultural and the industrial sectors, and in essential-service areas such as education and health. The health system may already be over-burdened and resources may be scarce. Even in a country that is coping, the emergency may be all it takes to turn a low-prevalence into a high-prevalence situation.

HIV can worsen the emergency situation by:

- Reducing resistance to disease in those already affected – through lack of food, lack of medication, and increased stress levels
- Undermining existing positive coping strategies in HIV-affected households, and over-burdening carers
- Placing more demand on resources (such as water supply in camps or shelters) for those who are HIV-positive and showing symptoms of AIDS (chronically ill) and their carers
- Making it difficult to find healthy workers for prevention programmes in camps; carers may not be free to take up volunteer posts or participate in cash for work programmes
- Causing the host community or other cultures and ethnic groups to discriminate against PLWHA in the new environment
- Increasing the vulnerability of orphans and other vulnerable children affected by HIV (OVCs), old people, and child-headed households, due to the fact that they may have difficulty in getting food, may be last in the line to receive scarce rations, and may not be able to collect water and firewood

Stembile says:

Be prepared! You need to know about the pre-emergency situation in your country. How did HIV affect the population before the emergency?

2.4 Vulnerable groups

In a humanitarian emergency there will be certain factors such as age, gender, social disability, and HIV status that affect vulnerability and people's ability to cope with the disaster. The Sphere Project defines key vulnerable groups as women, children, older people, disabled people, PLWHA, and ethnic minorities. These same groups have been used here for consistency. First we review the susceptibility of these groups to HIV infection and then we look at how an emergency situation can make this worse for each group.

2.4.1 Women and girls

These are the factors that increase the susceptibility of women and girls to HIV infection:

- **Physiological:** the virus is found in greater concentration in semen than in vaginal secretions so women are more likely to get infected by men than men are by women. In addition, tearing and bleeding during intercourse, whether from rough sex, rape, or prior genital mutilation (female circumcision), increases infection risk.

- **Social:** In many countries, women are often not in a position to negotiate when it comes to sexual matters, and there may be stereo-typing of 'loose women' (the assumption that because a woman agrees to sex once, she is immoral or is therefore a commercial sex worker). Many societies tolerate multiple partners in men but not in women. Young girls may be brought up with lit-tle sexual or reproductive health knowledge, making them even more vulnerable to infections.

- **Economic:** Women who lack economic resources may be more accepting of violent sexual behaviour if they fear that their partner may abandon them if they refuse. The phenomenon of 'sugar daddies' where older men pay young girls for sex (often in kind) occurs in many developing countries. (See Box 4.)

2.4.2 Young males

These are the factors that increase the susceptibility of men and especially young boys to HIV infection:[14]

- Social norms that reinforce their lack of understanding of sexual health issues and their toleration of promiscuity

- Substance abuse such as drugs or alcohol, which may lead to prostitution or simply sex for subsistence (sex tourism)[15]

- Sex for subsistence (without substance abuse), which may be an alternative in times of hardship

- Types of work that can entail mobility and family disruption (migrant labour, truck driving, fishing, and military service)

Box 4: Sex for subsistence

Commercial sex workers have often been called an important 'core group' and sometimes have even been labelled the principal 'vectors' of the AIDS epidemic.[13] This accusation has resulted in further stigmatisation. Prostitution in many developing countries is an imprecise term as some women, who would not classify themselves as sex workers, use sex as payment for favours (often in lieu of paying bills) or to supplement meagre incomes – a phenomenon usually referred to as sex for subsistence.

Women may turn to commercial sex work or sex for subsistence as an alternative to poverty, or because their lives have been disrupted by war, divorce, or widowhood where, because of inequitable laws and customs, they have lost their property and their husband's earnings. As one Zimbabwean woman said:

'It is better to get AIDS than to watch your kids starving.'

The group of (usually) women who use sex for subsistence are the hardest to reach, as it is often a secret arrangement linked to feelings of guilt and shame. These women seldom consider themselves to be sex workers and because they depend on the sexual transactions for survival, they are not in a position to negotiate for protection.

An example of sex for subsistence

In Zimbabwe where the economic crisis and rampant inflation has increased the number of people living below the poverty line, more women may be forced to turn to sex for subsistence. Agnes is a single mother with two children living in a rural community after her husband left her for another woman. She admits to having one boyfriend who buys her food and another who pays her children's school fees. She is adamant that she is not a sex worker but admits that she cannot use a condom when sleeping with her boyfriends as 'it would be looking like I am ungrateful for his help'.

2.4.3 Effect of an emergency on women and girls and young males

- In conflict there is increased risk of rape, sexual abuse, or pressure to engage in sexual favours by armed forces and displaced men
- In conflict there may be forced recruitment of child soldiers (both male and female)
- In times of drought or deprivation, sex for subsistence may increase
- Boredom in camps may lead to increased drug and alcohol abuse with possible unprotected sex as a consequence
- A lack of role models and family support may lead to more promiscuity and unprotected sex

Box 5 gives an example of one way to work with young people.

Box 5: An example of working with young people

In country X during a drought response, health promoters doing house-to-house visits found that young girls were reluctant to leave their houses, due to problems with the availability of sanitary materials. Whilst talking about these issues, the promoters were able to open the discussion to a more general one around sexual health and HIV and AIDS. Later, groups included young boys who also needed more information and a chance to ask questions. This work was an integral part of the hygiene promotion but was a response to felt needs by young people in the drought-affected area. As the humanitarian programme was time-bound, this particular aspect of the programme was handed on to a local NGO who could expand the activities.

2.4.4 The elderly, the disabled, and ethnic minorities

There are a growing number of elderly people taking care of small children either due to the death of a parent or because parents have migrated to seek work. In a high-prevalence country, there may be no grown-up children to care for elderly parents, who are left to fend for themselves. An elderly carer who was already looking after a disabled person may suddenly find themselves caring for orphans as well.

Effect of an emergency on this group

In an emergency families and communities may become separated. Elderly and disabled people are often left on their own, without their families, and this can lead to exploitation and abuse that can expose them to HIV.

Disabled people may be exploited or neglected if they have special needs that are difficult to meet during the emergency; for example a visually impaired person may have to use communal latrines that have not been adapted to make it easier for that person to use.

Being a member of an ethnic minority does not in itself lead to greater susceptibility to HIV infection, but marginalisation due to ethnicity may limit access to services and resources.

2.4.5 People living with HIV and AIDS (PLWHA)

In developing countries, a large percentage of HIV-positive people may never be tested and will therefore not consider themselves to be vulnerable. Even if people do know their status, they may not admit it, because there is always a possibility that they will be stigmatised and discriminated against by the rest of the society. This may result in divorce or loss of employment or in the person being forced to leave home. Despite the fact that several prominent people have been open about being HIV-positive, in reality they are the minority.

Effect of an emergency on this group

Lack of medical services, especially access to antibiotics and anti-retrovirals, will seriously affect the health of HIV-positive people. They may develop AIDS more quickly than they would in a non-emergency situation. Lack of food, clean water, and general hygienic facilities will all have a harmful effect on the health of this group. Disruption and displacement may lead to separation of the infected person and their carer.

The carer may be absent for much of the day if they are taking part in cash for work or have to queue for rations. The ill person will have no-one to feed them or to attend to their bodily needs.

Discrimination may occur if someone is suspected of being HIV-positive, especially among displaced people in a host community. Known HIV-positive people may also be stigmatised if it is felt that they and their families are getting more aid than others (see page 25).

Stembile says:

Consider the needs both of people infected by HIV and those affected by it!

Avoid stigmatisation and discrimination!

Section 3:
How to mainstream HIV and AIDS in emergencies

This section gives advice about mainstreaming throughout the emergency project cycle. The project cycle has been divided into the following phases:

- 3.1 Pre-emergency preparedness
- 3.2 Assessment
- 3.3 Implementation
- 3.4 Monitoring and evaluation

3.1 Pre-emergency preparedness

3.1.1 Information gathering

One activity which helps in the preparedness phase is gathering specific information that helps map the susceptibility and vulnerability of a population to HIV and AIDS. Much of this kind of information can be found on websites or obtained from agencies such as the Ministry of Health, WHO, or UNDP.

The Country Specific Epidemiological Fact Sheets on HIV/AIDS (www.unaids.org) give a very broad indication of general levels and patterns of HIV prevalence within a country and provide the following information:

- Estimated numbers of PLWHA – disaggregated by gender and age
- Estimated deaths due to AIDS
- Estimated numbers of OVCs
- HIV sentinel surveillance information (sites where specific groups of people are routinely tested, such as university students)
- Curable STIs – incidence and prevalence

- Health Service Indicators including access to health care[16] and condom availability for both males and females

Also useful at this preparedness stage is information about:

- Population (if at all feasible, disaggregated by gender and age)
- Other agencies (local, national, international) working in HIV prevention and treatment
- Partner preparedness and capacity
- The government HIV and AIDS policy and programmes, including awareness programmes
- The availability of antiretrovirals and costings
- The level of acceptance and availability of testing services
- The religious community's attitude to HIV and AIDS, and especially to condoms

Stembile says:

Remember many people in developing countries don't know their status and therefore they are never included in official statistics. The fact sheets only give an idea of what the trends may be like – treat them with caution.

3.2 Assessment

3.2.1 Questions to ask

This HIV and AIDS assessment should be part of a general public health assessment and situational analysis. Try not to collect too much extra information at this stage but use the general vulnerability criteria (from the Sphere Project – see page 13 – as well as chronically ill) to capture data on potential PLWHA. Here are some suggested questions to ask:

• Are health services still functioning and what do they provide for people who are HIV-positive?

• Are other agency interventions addressing the social, medical, protection, education, or human rights aspects of HIV and AIDS? Is there a service for antiretrovirals, post exposure prophylaxis (PEP),[17] and counselling?

• Are condoms available and what is the distribution mechanism?

• What is the situation with trucking (water, food, and non-food items)? Are there many non-local truck drivers staying in the area?

• Are there foreign peacekeepers and are they from a high-prevalence country?

• Has there been an influx of refugees and what is the prevalence rate in the country from which they are coming?

• Has the situation increased the population's contact with armed groups?

• What HIV prevention and care facilities were available in the country of origin and what facilities are available now?

• Are the project staff knowledgeable about HIV and AIDS and the Code of Conduct?[18]

• What are the primary diseases and infections? (Disaggregate data by gender and age.[19] Remember that Tuberculosis [TB] rates can be an indicator for HIV- infected persons.)

• Are any health promotion initiatives or activities taking place?

- Are there any local structures with whom you could collaborate in health promotion activities?
- Have available health promoters or community health workers had previous education or experience in STIs and HIV?

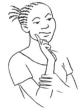

Stembile says:

Remember that proxy indicators such as increased STI rates, TB, and chronic illness can give you an idea about the prevalence of HIV and AIDS, but be careful of stigmatising anyone suffering from these.

3.2.2 Methods for collecting information

There are no special methods for collecting information about HIV and AIDS. Mainstreaming means using the methods you would normally use but thinking about the possibility that there may be HIV-positive people, AIDS patients, and their carers among the primary stakeholders. All participatory rural appraisal (PRA) methods can be adapted.[20] The important thing is not to assume that anyone is HIV-positive, and to avoid stigmatisation. The broader the range of people with whom you consult, the greater the chance of you actually talking to those affected or infected. Remember that people who are HIV-positive may not attend meetings or focus groups if they feel they are being singled out – to avoid this make sure people are invited to meetings to talk about general problems rather than AIDS.

You can also use the Scoring Tool on page 24 to look at specific potential risks for the country you are working in.

Stembile Suggestion

In a focus group with women, you may want to talk about the possibility of increased sex for subsistence. It could be very sensitive and embarrassing, so instead you could

say: 'people say that more women are being paid for sex in order to survive in this emergency. Have you heard of anyone doing that in your community?'
See, a safe way to ask and very non-threatening!

3.2.3 Minimum response

One of the key aspects of mainstreaming HIV and AIDS is that there is *always* a minimum response. This can be summed up by 'do no harm' – trying to minimise the way in which your work may make people more susceptible to HIV infection (Holden 2004). Reducing opportunities for sexual and gender-based violence, and main-streaming gender issues (for example women's safety), as well as raising staff awareness will go a long way in achieving this goal. Especially in the acute phase of an emergency, this minimum approach is probably the most effective. Co-ordinating with other NGOs, national or local authorities, and local partners could also be part of the approach.

Stembile Suggestion

A quick checklist for minimum response is:

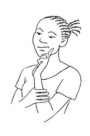

    Keep the focus of your humanitarian programme
    Avoid stigmatisation – use vulnerable households or chronically
        ill as criteria
    Find out about the HIV and AIDS situation in the emergency-
        affected country
    In water and sanitation work, consider the safety and
        protection of vulnerable groups
    Make sure your staff are informed about HIV facts
    Livelihoods work should be suited to the special needs of both
        those affected and infected
    Consider issues of gender and protection
    Make sure that there is good two-way communication and flow
        of information between the emergency-affected community
        and your organisation

3.2.4 A scoring tool for managers and planners

By using the scoring tool below, the manager and the team can determine the likelihood of increased transmission and vulnerability of the affected population. This tool can be used both in proposal writing and in planning the programme. For every yes answer, score one. For every no answer, score zero. The higher the total score, the more urgent is the need for HIV mainstreaming. However, you do need also to look at **which** of the factors increases the risk – is it the fact that it is refugees from a high-prevalence country or is it the presence of foreign troops? See the Aceh example in Box 6 opposite.

Question	Answer		Score
Is there a high HIV prevalence in the country or region of refugee/IDP origin?	Yes	No	
Is there a high HIV prevalence in the country or region of operation?	Yes	No	
Has there been displacement of people into camps or shelters?	Yes	No	
Has there been increased migration of people out of their own area because of the emergency?	Yes	No	
Are there mobile men such as contractors, truck drivers, or casual labourers in the programme area?	Yes	No	
Are there national/foreign troops present?	Yes	No	
Is there a large number of foreign aid workers present?	Yes	No	
Is there an increased risk of sexual abuse?	Yes	No	
Is there a shortage of food (resulting in potential for sex for subsistence)?	Yes	No	
Is there a lack of government openness to HIV and support to prevention programmes?[21]	Yes	No	
Is there a low uptake for voluntary counselling and testing (VCT) services among the affected population? (Shows lack of openness and awareness)	Yes	No	

There will be mitigating factors to take into account as well, such as community support and cultural norms regarding the protection of single women. These will vary from country to country but will usually be known to national staff or community-based organisations.

Box 6: An example of using the scoring tool

Although Aceh province in Indonesia is an isolated area in a low-prevalence country (1 out of 1000 adults aged 15–49 are estimated to be infected in the whole of Indonesia, according to UNAIDS), the score during the 2005 tsunami response was actually 7, when using the Scoring Tool above. Despite the province (which is predominantly Muslim) being cut off from the rest of the world for so long, the tsunami brought huge changes such as an influx of foreign workers (and diaspora Acehnese) and military personnel. There was also an increased risk of sexual abuse, with people living in temporary camps sharing sanitation and bathing facilities, as well as a general lack of awareness about HIV and a reluctance to talk about sexual matters. However, the mitigating factors are the cultural norms for sexual behaviour and the strong community cohesiveness. The score would show a manager that the areas of concern for the programme would be women's safety, HIV and Code of Conduct training for staff, and making sure that any suspected sexual abuse by troops or aid workers is addressed.

3.2.5 Stigmatisation and how to avoid it

UNAIDS estimates that more than 90 per cent of HIV-positive people do not know their status. Even those that do know may not necessarily disclose this information to others, as they may be afraid of being marginalised or even discriminated against both socially and in the workplace. Stigmatisation in its many forms isolates people and denies them their basic human rights.

Even in non-emergency situations, the following can occur:

- National policy and laws can create stigma (such as mandatory testing, and acceptance of HIV-positive people losing their jobs because of their status).
- Unless access to antiretrovirals is free, those too poor to afford treatment or without the means to travel to heath facilities face discrimination.

- Families can reject a family member who discloses their status, leaving the person alone and without family support.
- Certain groups such as commercial sex workers and homosexuals are blamed for the spread of HIV.
- Lack of insurance policies or redundancy packages for people who lose their jobs through discrimination or illness can leave them destitute.

No matter what form it takes, stigmatisation is detrimental to prevention, care, and treatment of HIV and AIDS. Organisations can work to end stigmatisation by helping people gain access to information on their rights and by advocating for this at the local, national, and international levels. Information on human rights should be available in the local language for all staff, as a first step to stop discrimination.

It should be remembered that HIV-positive people are fit and healthy until they begin to show signs of opportunistic infections. Even then, with the right treatment they can be involved in communal activities suited to their physical abilities. However, this may not be understood either by staff or by other beneficiaries.

Targeting humanitarian relief to households affected by HIV and AIDS can increase stigma and exclusion unless done sensitively and with the full participation of those **infected** and **affected**. The best way to avoid stigmatisation is simply to target all households where there are chronically ill people, because if HIV prevalence is high, there is a chance that those people are ill due to AIDS. Vulnerability of a particular household can be worked out using the ratio of well carers to unwell family members. The higher the ratio of dependants to carer, the harder it will be for carers to cope, especially if they are elderly, or children, or are themselves unwell. You may want to work out this ratio during nutritional surveys or when you are registering for hygiene kit distribution.

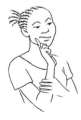

Stembile Suggestion
If there are local trusted NGOs already working with HIV-affected or infected families, work with them.

3.3 Implementation

In every humanitarian programme, there will be different sectors involved. In a typical Oxfam response for example, there will be water, sanitation, and hygiene promotion, livelihoods and possibly shelter. There will also be cross-cutting issues such as gender, accountability, and advocacy to consider. All these areas will be addressed here.

3.3.1 Water, sanitation, and public health promotion

As in any public health emergency, provision of adequate water and sanitation facilities will promote and maintain good health. One of the common causes of diarrhoea is poor water quality and lack of sanitation. Diarrhoea is one of the common complaints suffered by people with HIV and AIDS, and when chronic, can lead quickly to debilitation.

HIV and AIDS mainstreamed interventions are not very different from those proposed for gender-based violence interventions, generally vulnerable groups, or protection programmes. In other words, most of the following points are just good programming:

- Consult with women and children on the siting of latrines, bathing areas, and areas provided for washing and drying menstrual cloths

- Remember that those caring for sick people may not have the time to attend meetings – house to house visits are more appropriate

- Provide safe and (if possible) well-lit latrines, water points, and washing facilities in order to prevent sexual attacks. If candles and lamps are a fire hazard, consider solar lighting or handheld solar lamps

- Consider family latrines or shared family latrines (several families to one latrine)

- Consider having more latrines for women, as women tend to use latrines more frequently than men and are normally in charge of children's hygiene

- Train water and sanitation committees so that they understand HIV issues and the needs of those affected or infected in terms of sanitation and access to water
- Make sure that 50 per cent of water committees are female so that women's safety will be a priority
- Consider the fact that some of the water and sanitation committee may be AIDS-affected, and illness may be an issue. Be prepared for drop-outs and re-trainings during the life of the programme
- Consider the 'out-of-sight' needs of chronically ill and bedridden people within the camp, including those with AIDS. They may need an increased amount of water for washing due to fever, vomiting, and diarrhoea
- Consider assistance in gathering water, or special deliveries of water to bedridden people, as carers may be unable both to look after sick people and collect adequate amounts of water. If this is not possible, consider providing extra jerricans both for collection and storage
- Install a hand pump where the handle does not go too high when released – otherwise children have to jump to get it down again. Most modern hand pumps are child-friendly but it is always good to check
- Check regularly that the foot valve is functioning, otherwise it is very hard for children, older people, or those weakened by disease to pump
- Provide a windlass on open wells instead of a bucket and rope
- Give out five-litre collapsible jerricans for children, as they are easier to carry
- Consider treadle pumps for easy use – see Figure 2

Figure 2: A treadle pump adapted for use by people with reduced strength

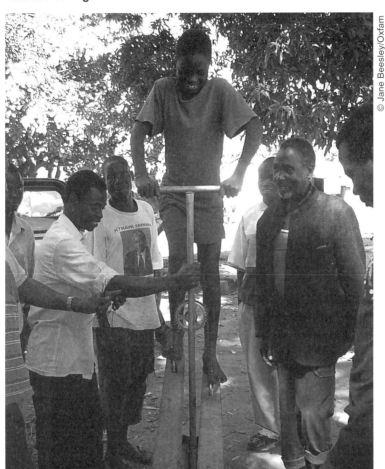

These pumps are in the community of Kapichi in Thyolo District, Malawi.
They were funded by NOVIB for an Oxfam International Project.

Stembile says:

If possible, make the water points child and elderly friendly!

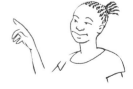

Box 8: An example of HIV mainstreaming in water projects

In Kitgum in Northern Uganda, some IDP camp communities agreed that those families with a chronically ill member would be exempt from paying water user fees. The community water user group also agreed that those families could jump the queue at the water points in order to reduce waiting time, thereby allowing them to collect more water.

Adapt latrines to make them more user-friendly for those who are weakened by infections (and for elderly carers or children) by providing:

- Wooden rather than metal lids, as metal lids are heavy and can cause damage if dropped on toes or feet
- A ramp instead of steps, if the latrine is raised
- A bar to hold when squatting, or a seat (see Figures 3 and 4)

These and further ideas can be found in the book *Water and sanitation for disabled people and other vulnerable groups; designing service to improve accessibility* (Jones and Reed 2005).

Figure 3: Moveable wooden ramp   Figure 4: Toilet stool

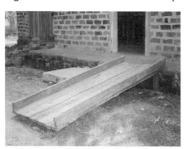 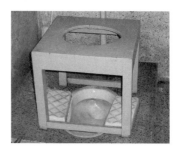

© Jones and Reed 2005,
used with permission.

© Jones and Reed 2005,
used with permission.

3.3.2 Information, education, and condom distribution (IEC)

Information

In development programmes, PLWHA can often play a crucial role in informing people about HIV and AIDS, but this is difficult in an emergency setting unless there is a local group or NGO for PLWHA which could assist.

Here are some points to be aware of when communicating about HIV and AIDS:[22]

- Although it is good to give out information, do not just add on a message about HIV to general public health messages. Behaviour change is more complicated than just providing information, and printing a poster or T-shirt with an AIDS message is probably a waste of time unless an effort is made to follow up either on an individual or small group basis.

- Do not be negative. Do not use images of death or skeletons to illustrate the end result of HIV infection. There is no evidence that this has ever changed behaviour. In an emergency, risk-taking and death from HIV and AIDS can be seen as secondary to the immediate disaster – as in East Timor, where one staff member commented: 'if you have lived through 1999 and saw your family die, why should death from AIDS be anything to be worried about? It could almost be a relief'. Make the messages positive: protect your family and stay healthy, for example.

- Provide information on HIV and AIDS in an integrated way that is culturally appropriate – for example in a focus group discussing protection issues with women in a camp.

- Use a credible source – use people who are respected in their community (such as a nurse or a head teacher) to communicate the message.

- Capture the audience's attention – make them feel part of the problem and the solution.

- Address the gender dimensions of the epidemic but do not portray women as victims.

- Promote gender equity and human rights.
- Touch the heart as well as the mind of the audience – make them feel that the message addresses them directly, and use the active rather than the passive voice.
- Make the message relevant and related to real life – this is especially important in emergencies, where options may not be possible.
- Ask the audience to take action, and provide realistic options for behaviour change.
- Surprise the audience – make it fresh, unusual, and original.

The 'right' message can also be misunderstood. In the Zambia 2002/2003 food crisis, well-meaning staff, eager to mainstream, painted red ribbons on all the trucks distributing food. Communities interpreted this as meaning that the food was destined for PLWHA only.

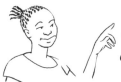

Stembile says:

Check out all messages with the community first!

Education

Make sure that carers of chronically ill people understand the importance of cleanliness and proper disposal of infected matter from open wounds or vomit, urine, or stools where there is blood (see Box 9).

Do not assume that people with education have a good understanding of HIV and other STI transmission – make sure you know their level of understanding and check for misconceptions.

Box 9: An example of HIV mainstreaming in public health promotion

In camp X, the public health promoters reported that there were several families with chronically ill adults who required varying degrees of nursing care. The team leader contacted a local NGO already working with PLWHA and together they visited the families to discuss with them what Oxfam could do to help. The main problem seemed to be that the ill person suffered from chronic diarrhoea, among other symptoms. The team leader agreed that the family needed two extra jerricans as they were using a great deal of water, and Oxfam would also supply a container to be used as a bedpan. It was explained to the family the necessity for strict cleanliness of this utensil and how the contents must be emptied down the pit latrine. The public health promoters made bi-weekly monitoring visits to check on how things were going. These visits were combined with their normal house to house visits, so did not take up any extra time.

Condoms and other preventive measures

In non-emergency situations, the three messages of abstinence, be faithful, and use a condom have been used to prevent transmission through sexual intercourse. It is important that programmes give out information in order that people can make a choice, rather than advocating for one message that may be against the beliefs of the beneficiaries.

Abstinence – this implies that people have a choice. However, in many cases women of all ages are not given the choice in sexual relations: they may be forced by their partners or, as occurs in many emergencies, raped by other people. Rape of men does happen but is much more stigmatised, and less likely to be discussed.

Be faithful – this implies that both partners can remain faithful to each other. In many cultures men have partners outside of marriage (women do as well but it is not widely reported), while their partners may be faithful. This puts one partner at risk of infection. If families are separated either by force or by the necessity of seeking work elsewhere, men may find new sexual partners, either casual or semi-permanent ones. In IDP or refugee situations, sex for subsistence may be the only livelihood alternative for women.

Use a condom – according to the Inter-Agency Standing Committee Guidelines for HIV Interventions in Emergency Settings, 'one of the most urgent tasks facing emergency relief agencies during acute phase is to make condoms freely available to those who seek them. This includes relief workers' (IASC 2004: 68). In addition, female condoms should be made available to populations who are used to them.

In reality the situation is far more complex. Condoms are a controversial issue in most environments and need to be dealt with in a sensitive and appropriate way. There are cultural and religious issues to be considered before launching into condom distribution as the key preventive measure in an emergency. Aid agencies cannot make choices for people – we can give information and resources but the choice has to be up to individuals (see Box 10). Here are some key things to consider when doing condom distribution:

- Do not give out condoms without doing preliminary assessment or discussing with communities – it can be offensive to some religions, people may not know how to use them, and in some instances distribution could give the wrong message (forced sex is OK if you just use a condom).

- Discuss with the primary stakeholders (the community members, displaced persons, or refugees benefiting from the programme) the best way to give out condoms, whether it is appropriate to distribute both male and female condoms, and where people would like to go to get them.

- Women often do not have the power to negotiate condom use with partners, so it is worth linking up with a peer-education programme or a prevention programme that works with women on developing negotiation skills.

Stembile Suggestion

In a country where condoms are less accepted, choose some
key people in the camp or in the community who are willing
to keep condoms. These could be community health workers,
traditional birth attendants, or community leaders.
Check to make sure there are no concerns from the local
religious leaders or government health services. During
health discussions with the community, they can be told
where condoms are available but also be told about
abstinence and faithfulness. They can then make a choice.

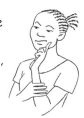

Box 10: An example of working with high-risk groups

Truck drivers are considered a high-risk group because of their being mostly
male and very mobile. They often spend nights away from home and are at
risk of infection from casual sex in overnight stops. Think about giving them
some information and condoms. In Zambia during the food crisis, Oxfam was
using trucks to bring in food. The truck drivers spent many hours on the road
and often slept in guesthouses along the way. A leaflet explaining about HIV
and AIDS, awareness sessions, and condoms were offered to all drivers
before they set off on their journeys. They were also given condoms and
leaflets to distribute to other drivers, which they did successfully. The drivers
also provided condoms to truck stops and petrol stations along their route.
Big signs were put up: condoms available here.

Stembile says:

Mainstreaming should never just be an add-on to pacify
donors or managers – rather it should be happening
because we think we can make a difference and
mitigate or prevent the spread of HIV.

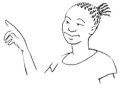

3.3.3 Shelter

Single women and child-headed households may be vulnerable to sexual abuse and therefore they need to know that their living quarters are safe from intruders, especially at night. This may be difficult in an acute situation when people are living in tents or small shelters. However, you might consider:

• Arranging shelter for IDPs with close family or community members

• Suggesting that single women live together in groups

• Placing child-headed households near people who can be trusted – older women, for example

See Box 11 for two examples of HIV mainstreaming in shelter programmes.

Box 11: Examples of HIV mainstreaming in shelter programmes

In Sri Lanka, when transitional houses were being built, the community asked for the units to be joined so that people would feel more secure. Locks were provided for the doors. This is an ideal situation for single women and child-headed households as well as those nursing chronically ill people.

In Northern Uganda in Kitgum town, there is the phenomenon of night dwellers: children who live in villages around the town but who walk into town at night to sleep in buildings and outhouses in order to avoid being kidnapped by a rebel faction called the Lord's Resistance Army. There is a huge potential for HIV spread due to the mixing of sexes and the vulnerability of small children sleeping in unprotected and unsupervised places. Oxfam and other NGOs have built shelters for these children with separate rooms for girls, with well-lit latrines and with a fence. A national NGO is carrying out awareness sessions with the children.

3.3.4 Food security, livelihoods, and nutrition

The severity of food insecurity is measured by people's ability to feed themselves, based on:

- The availability of and access to food

- Their nutritional status – if people are undernourished before a food crisis there is a greater risk of them dying from hunger

- The impact on self-sufficiency in terms of production and creating income (risk to livelihoods)

From the onset of any emergency response it is important to attempt to integrate both the traditionally 'short-term' approach (concerned with saving lives through immediate aid, e.g. food distribution/feeding programmes or cash-transfer programmes[23]) and the 'longer-term' livelihood support involving interventions supporting the rehabilitation and/or recovery of livelihoods, e.g. animal restocking or seeds distribution.

This section covers nutrition and utilisation of food, and goes on to outline some strategies to address food insecurity.

Nutrition and HIV and AIDS

There are two levels at which HIV and AIDS and the nutritional status of the affected/infected family or individuals are linked:

1   The nutritional status of families and HIV-affected individuals can be altered by reduced income sources (loss of workforce due to illness) and/or different food sharing patterns within the households (main share of food is for those infected with HIV).

2   The infected individual has to cope not only with a possible reduced availability of food but also a changed metabolism and digestion. Food intake may be decreased due to poor appetite or mouth infections, nutrient malabsorption, metabolic alterations, and frequent diarrhoea, whilst at the same time increased energy requirements are often observed.[24]

It is important to remember that micronutrients play an increasingly important role in HIV-infected individuals[25] – for example:

- Vitamins A, B6, and B12, iron, zinc, and selenium build and maintain a strong immune system[26] and fight infections
- Lack of Vitamin A is associated with higher mother-to-child transmission rates, faster progression from HIV to AIDS, and higher infant mortality and child growth failure
- B-group vitamins play important roles in maintaining a healthy immune system and hindering progression of HIV and AIDS

Utilisation of food

Nutritionally balanced and hygienically prepared food is important but equally so is the intra-household distribution of food which may not always favour those who need it most (because of the custom of men eating first, children sharing a plate, stronger children eating more). All intervention activities should always include some education and awareness-raising about good nutritional and feeding practices. This is not just for HIV-positive people but also for all vulnerable groups in an emergency. Here are some ideas for how to do this in practice:

- Provide information on good utilisation, preparation, and storage of foods. Provide resources (utensils and information) to encourage good practices.
- Work with communities to investigate all options for obtaining nutrients and promote local food habits that improve the intake of root vegetables, local vegetables and fruits, nuts, insects, oilseeds, and other wild foods that may add vital nutrients to the diet.
- Provide educational materials on nutrition and feeding practices to ensure that PLWHA maintain a healthy diet, manage illness, and monitor and maintain their nutritional status. Especially work on how to relieve eating difficulties through natural remedies and food preparations (FAO/WHO 2002).

These ideas are of course fully workable in the ideal situation, whereas in many emergencies where rations are limited, the whole community is vulnerable.

Mother-to-child transmission and breast-feeding

'Breast is best' has always been promoted by development and humanitarian agencies, encouraging mothers to breast-feed their babies for at least the first four to six months.[27] However, breast-feeding is associated with increased risks of HIV transmission from mother to child. Therefore the UN IASC Guidelines (IASC 2004) suggest that breast-feeding should be avoided whenever replacement feeding (bottle feeding with formula milk) is **acceptable, feasible, affordable, sustainable, and safe.** But in emergency settings, the risk of babies dying from diarrhoea is often greater than the risk of HIV transmission, and being able to keep bottles and other utensils clean and safe is often simply not an option.

Recent studies have shown that the risk of infection can be reduced by **exclusive** breast-feeding for the first four to six months with a **very short** (a couple of days) weaning period at the end of the six months.[28] However, WHO states that exclusive breast-feeding for the 'first few months' is recommended, with weaning over a 'few days to a few weeks'.[29]

Access to food

Every situation needs to be carefully assessed and an analysis carried out to make sure that affected families' members and infected individuals are getting enough food. In order to support the affected households most appropriately, it is necessary to consider both the access to food and the availability and utilisation of food.

If the access to food is the reason for inadequate food intake (due to insufficient income), a cash-transfer programme to the affected/infected households (for example by providing cash for work) could be the appropriate strategy in an emergency situation. This would increase purchasing power and ensure well-balanced and adequate food intake, but only if food is available on local markets. Ensuring that a valid livelihoods initiative does not inadvertently increase the risk of HIV transmission is an important part of mainstreaming (see Box 12).

Box 12: An example of a programme potentially affecting the prevalence rates

In Turkana district in Kenya, a team of field staff were visiting a village during a routine monitoring trip. Whilst walking around and observing, they talked to several women who, when asked what sickness there was in the village, replied that some houses had very thin, very sick people. It turned out that these houses were the homes of men who had left the village to work in a nearby town. Away from their families and with money in their pockets, they paid for sex and subsequently contracted HIV. The team realised that their cash for work programme, where village men were paid to do bush clearance near the town, could expose these men to an increased risk of contracting the virus.

Availability of food

If it is the availability of food which is the problem, various strategies could be considered. These are outlined below:

• In any situation, a general food ration can be provided to families who are food insecure. Specially identified vulnerable households[30] could receive a supplementary food ration, which needs to be complementary to the distribution of a general food ration. Beware of possible stigmatisation with this distribution.

• In many situations, including camps, shelters, or community-based programmes, selected vulnerable groups could be provided with a special prepared diet to ensure minimum intake of food. A distribution of special food components could be considered: fresh vegetables, animal protein (e.g. eggs/milk), and fruits are examples.

• If you are not working for the agency responsible for food distribution, consider advocating for additional nutrient supplement in food distribution where HIV prevalence is high. This is only likely to have any impact where the general ration is adequate.[31]

There will be situations when providing food aid is not an appropriate or the most sensitive response:

- When the risk of stigmatising PLWHA or affected households through food distribution is high. The advantages and disadvantages will have to be considered.
- When individuals or affected households are able to meet their own food needs.
- When cash is more appropriate than food.
- When available foods for food aid are inappropriate for dietary needs or cultural conditions.

Stembile Suggestion

Use the criteria of OVCs, child-headed households, elderly people without support, and households with chronically ill people in them. This way you won't stigmatise those who may possibly be infected with HIV. Be careful about combining HIV and AIDS education messages and food distribution in case people think the messages are targeting potentially infected households.

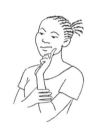

Box 13: An example of HIV mainstreaming in livelihoods programmes – gardens

Even in space-restricted areas such as camps, micro-gardening can be done – either in small plots around the tent/house or at communal grounds. If it is performed on an individual basis for each house, consider trees that might supply natural remedies assisting digestion and relieving other symptoms. Papaya trees are one example: they mature fast and are good for healing lesions and ulcers in the mouth as well as supporting protein digestion. Vegetables are an important food source as well as being an added source of income with surplus sale. In establishing a garden, the distance from the house is important, as carers may need to attend both to the sick person and to the garden – so ensure minimal walking time. Community gardens have the advantage of sharing working time among various families in the management of the garden. Any activities should contain a good training on cultivation techniques, vegetable varieties and use, and possibly some marketing ideas.

Food production

Food production leading to self-sufficiency could be considered in some humanitarian situations but is dependent on local conditions and seasonality. For infected/affected households, consider either low labour input or shared labour activities:

- **Home and community gardens:** the diet can be improved through eating varied foods, and selling surplus can provide a valuable cash source to support other household and individual needs. There are also some specific foods that are beneficial for opportunistic infections and examples of these can be found in the FAO Nutrition manual (FAO/WHO 2002) (see Box 13 and Figure 5).

- **Agricultural support:** crop diversification can ensure a wide range of adequate and fresh foods for consumption and surplus sale, and introduce fast-maturing and low labour-intensive crop varieties and better cultivation techniques, which increase available caring time for family members of chronically ill individuals.

- **Small livestock:** raising small animals (chickens, rabbits, guinea pigs) helps improve the consumption of high quality protein, fat, iron, and Vitamin A. It is also an easy, low labour-intensive and less time-consuming source of income than growing crops. Good animal husbandry and cage/stable management is necessary to avoid exposure to infections in immuno-suppressed people, and the possibility of avian influenza needs to be considered in some countries (see Box 14).

- **Income-generating activities** should take account of the reduced capacity to work, both of those people infected and at the stage of not being able to carry out normal duties, and those who are caring for the ill. For carers, this may mean having an activity that takes into account nursing duties or care of orphans and children affected by the HIV epidemic.

See Box 15 on page 44 for more ideas of how to mainstream HIV in livelihoods programmes.

Figure 5: Community gardens in Zimbabwe

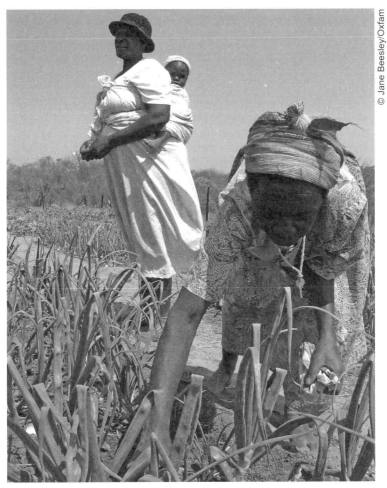

Cheziya Garden is a vegetable garden funded by Oxfam and the UK's
Department for International Development.

Box 14: The Chicken and egg story

Five vaccinated chicks (six weeks old, four female, one male) were distributed to identified households in country X. The targeting criteria used were: households with female or adolescent heads and chronically ill household members. Training on good animal husbandry and product management (e.g. eggs and meat) was included as part of the distribution package. Also provided were materials for a good cage, to reduce risk of infection to immuno- suppressed people, to provide a place for laying eggs, and to protect the new assets from poaching or wild animals. Monitoring activities showed that the chickens were a good choice to support the affected households because:

- Chickens don't need much care and can roam freely during the day, leaving time for carers to take care of household members, without reducing time to create income
- Chicken and eggs provide a good source of additional high-quality protein and income source from sale of surplus
- Chickens have a quick reproduction cycle which enables easy increase of animals per household

NB: The possibility of avian influenza needs to be taken into consideration and may make future chicken projects unacceptable.

Box 15: Further examples of mainstreaming in livelihoods
Small enterprises

In the IDP camps of Northern Kenya, women were trained to recycle plastic bags by making them into mats. The mats were woven and sold to the CARE water and sanitation sector for use in latrine-screening in the camps. Stronger women walked around the camp and collected up the bags, whilst those who were weaker worked at home or in the weaving centres. In two years, 2000 women made over $20,000 and helped remove 50 metric tons of plastic waste from the camps. The money was used to supplement food rations whilst some women started small-scale kiosks or bought goats.

Traditional herbs

In Zimbabwe, Oxfam worked to develop community gardens to increase micro-nutrients for beneficiary populations. The staff utilised local knowledge by consulting with a herbalist who knew the properties of the traditional plants and how to access the seeds. Local women and young people were organised to prepare the small plots of land and to plant and harvest the produce for their families. This can have a twofold benefit: 1) increase micronutrient consumption in vulnerable populations and 2) generate some income in areas where earning potential is difficult. Some plants have medicinal value for opportunistic infections.

Here are some other points to consider related to food security for the individual or at household level:

- Ensure minimisation of stigmatisation of individuals/households – see section on stigmatisation on page 25
- Discourage norms that deny women rations/cash or the right to inherit livestock and land
- Address security and environmental issues which decrease food security and livelihoods
- Enhance national capacity to manage food aid, food security, and livelihoods programmes

Stembile says:

Share the burden – involve communities in providing care and support to vulnerable households.

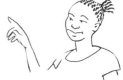

3.3.5 Cross-cutting issues: gender, protection, and accountability

Good programming integrates gender, protection, and HIV mainstreaming, as so many of the issues overlap. Good two-way communication underpins effective programming so that beneficiaries are informed about what to expect from the implementing agency and at the same time, programmes respond to changing needs as described by the affected communities (accountability). A good example is given in Box 16.

For further information in this area, refer to the Code of Good Practice for NGOs responding to HIV/AIDS.[32] Oxfam is a signatory to this code.

Box 16: An example of how to address cross-cutting issues in a programme

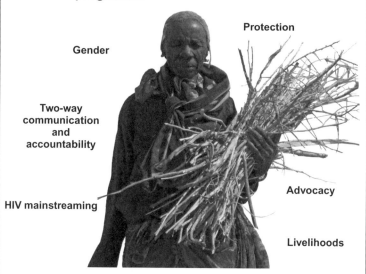

Gender

Protection

Two-way communication and accountability

HIV mainstreaming

Advocacy

Livelihoods

In the conflict in Darfur, women have been attacked and raped when they ventured outside the camps to collect firewood. As one leader said, the community had to make a choice: *'it is better for women to go to the field to look for sticks, grass, and firewood (either for sale or use in the house) than men because they will only be raped and abused and left to return while men will be killed'*.

This situation has implications for gender, protection, and HIV mainstreaming as well as being a violation of basic human rights.

Several agencies have started small projects to solve the firewood problem (livelihoods): lobbying for patrols to protect the women (advocacy and HIV mainstreaming), fuel-saving stove initiatives, and even the provision of fire-wood to the camps. Women can make and sell stoves, or sell the cooked food to earn a living, or simply use the wood to provide for their families.

Picture: A woman returns to Kalma camp for displaced people in South Darfur with a bundle of sticks to use for cooking.

© Adrian McIntyre/Oxfam

Stembile Suggestion

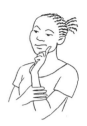

Starting a community discussion about a very practical issue can sometimes lead into more sensitive subjects. In the Democratic Republic of Congo (DRC), a focus group with women began by addressing their need for menstrual protection, which led the women to talk about rape and sexual violence.

3.4 Monitoring and evaluation

3.4.1 Overview

Monitoring is the systematic and continuous process of collecting and using information and presenting data, throughout the programme cycle, for the purpose of management and decision-making.

The indicators for measuring impact in HIV and AIDS prevention programmes are often HIV rates plus morbidity and mortality data. However, these changes occur over a long period and are not appropriate measures for humanitarian programmes as they entail sentinel surveillance (at pre-selected sites where groups such as university students are anonymously tested), reliable testing, and follow-up services such as counselling and antiretroviral therapy. Proxy indicators[33] such as gonorrhoea rates in men are often used instead.

Below are some example indicators for measuring the impact of HIV mainstreaming in public health promotion, water and sanitation, food security, and livelihoods programmes. There are both process[34] and impact[35] indicators for use at different stages of the programme.

3.4.2 Process indicators (how things are going)

Staff

- Number of staff who can name two ways in which the community may be susceptible to increased HIV transmission in the local context

- If appropriate – number of condoms distributed each month (disaggregated by men and women who ask for or receive condoms, if possible). This is a proxy indicator for condom use assuming that people are not selling them or supplying traders. If they are, this will tell you about the need for condoms rather than if staff are practising safe sex

Programme

The number of condoms distributed in the community could be used as a process indicator,[36] but it does not show whether these are being used and by whom. Better indicators are:

- Number of discussions had with individuals or community groups on HIV mainstreaming
- Number of vulnerable (chronic illness) households who express satisfaction with the facilities adapted for them
- Number of vulnerable (chronic illness) households who have received extra hygiene utensils
- Number of vulnerable (chronic illness) households using latrines
- Number of vulnerable households who state that they have received extra rations
- Number of vulnerable carers and child-headed households registered to receive extra food rations
- Number of female-headed households registered for cash for work programmes or livelihoods programmes

3.4.3 Impact indicators (what has happened as a result of mainstreaming)

Staff
- Number of staff who are able to state two ways in which they have mainstreamed HIV

Programme
- Number of women in a focus group who feel that they are protected from sexual harassment when using facilities
- Number of carers who express satisfaction with facilitated access to water and sanitation
- Number of vulnerable households who say that they have been dealt with in a dignified and caring manner in relation to ensuring that their needs are met by programme activities[37]

- Number of vulnerable households who state that there has been an improvement in the nutritional status of the chronically ill member since receiving extra rations
- Number of women in a focus group who can state examples where cash for work has reduced their susceptibility to HIV transmission

Stembile says:

HIV mainstreaming should be included at all stages of the project cycle – remember to put on those HIV glasses!

Section 4:
Advice for managers to help in planning

4.1 Internal (staff both national and international)

4.1.1 Who will be responsible for sharing information on HIV and AIDS?

Choose a person (or people) to be the designated HIV focal point for staff welfare. This person does not have to have a health-related role, but should be someone who is interested in the subject and has a genuine desire to provide information and support to their co-workers (see Box 17). It is best to have a man and a woman so that they can cover all gender aspects between them. Sometimes people in health-related roles hide behind the clinical jargon and may not feel comfortable talking about sensitive issues with other staff members. There is also the hierarchy to consider: drivers may not feel comfortable asking a manager for condoms or vice versa. Consider local culture and societal norms.

Box 17: Example of an HIV and AIDS focal point

In a country office, one person was chosen to be the HIV and AIDS focal point. The job included making sure there were condoms in the men's toilets (the women had opted for having condoms in a cupboard in the public health office), making sure all new staff were aware of HIV and AIDS mainstreaming, and finding out what facilities were available. The person made a list of all testing centres and surgeries which provided PEP and antiretrovirals, and NGOs involved in home-based care. When his colleague asked for help with her sick relative, he was able to point her in the right direction for assistance. The manager made sure that the focal point person had time to carry out his role.

4.1.2 How do I start doing something for my staff?

HIV and AIDS awareness training depends on the scale and nature of the emergency. Inductions should cover the minimum amount of information – see the activities and exercises in Section 5. Condoms can be provided after discussion with the staff about where they want them to be stored. Again, cultural considerations are important. In a high-risk country, trainings should start as soon as possible in order to reduce susceptibility and vulnerability.

4.1.3 What if a staff member confides that he/she is HIV-positive?

It can be a good idea to have a workplace policy based on the following guidelines:

- Make sure the person understands about confidentiality and that what they tell you will go no further. Also tell the person you will not write anything down.

- Take the lead from the infected person – they will know what information and assistance they require.

- Make sure the person knows what they have a right to, what services are available, and where to go for help.

- Remember, if the staff member wants to tell their colleagues about their status, they have a 'right to be heard'. Support them if this is what they want.

- Remember that there is no reason why someone can't continue working if they have no symptoms. It is only if they start to have periods of absenteeism due to illness, or become too tired or weak to carry out their work, that you will have to consider changing their role and responsibilities to suit their condition.

- If the person wants you to be their mentor and support them, think about whether you have the time and emotional energy to do this or whether it is better to find someone else for this role.

- Be aware of your own feelings about the situation and how they affect you. Feelings can rake up unresolved emotions from the past. Value these feelings because they may give you an insight into what both of you need and how you can best deal with the situation.

4.2 External (mainstreaming in the programme)

Use the scoring tool on page 24 to decide what the risks are for HIV transmission in your programme country.

Stembile says:

check back to look at the minimum response – is this what you need to do?

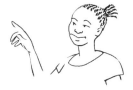

It is difficult to say exactly when it is appropriate to start HIV mainstreaming activities in a community; it will depend on the scale and rapidity of onset of the emergency and the nature of the response. However, once the immediate life-saving phase is over (for example once hygiene kits have been distributed and everyone has access to water and sanitation), there should be time for other activities. These could be:

- Community meetings and training of volunteers – see Section 5.
- Sectoral interventions – see Section 3.
- Advocacy and lobbying for services and access at co-ordination meetings.
- Setting up a system for whistle blowing – if staff members or community members witness or have information about sexual exploitation, they should be able to bring this to the attention of programme managers. However, people do need to beware of accusing anyone without evidence.

4.2.1 Frequently asked questions

1. *What is the point of worrying about HIV in a large-scale emergency when people have died of other causes and where epidemics are a real threat to survivors?*

   Of course, relief workers have to prioritise, and we may not start AIDS-awareness training in a first stage emergency. Oxfam, for example, has a mandate first and foremost to save lives. There is an obligation, however, after the acute phase, to consider the longer-term impact of the AIDS epidemic. This manual explains how to mainstream without detracting from other major health issues.

2. *Do I always have to mainstream HIV and AIDS even if my programme is in a low-prevalence country?*

Even in a low-prevalence country, managers should consider some form of HIV and AIDS mainstreaming. The minimum response is to make sure all staff are knowledgeable, condoms are available, and that the workplace policy is understood. It would be good to monitor the situation through the local Ministry of Health and through other medical NGOs working in the country.

3. *People already on antiretrovirals (drugs that slow the transition from HIV to AIDS) are often affected by an emergency when the drug supply chain is disrupted. Should a new chain be established by aid agencies?*

Supplying antiretrovirals means monitoring compliance, dosage, and side effects, which is best done through a clinical establishment. This must be done with a view to a longer-term commitment. In an emergency, Oxfam lobbies for other medical authorities or NGOs (with a proven track record in this area) to take on the task and to make sure that co-ordination bodies such as OCHA address the issue. Aid agencies can also assist with information-sharing and encouraging those affected to attend clinic sessions.

4. *Voluntary counselling and testing centres are a good way to help raise awareness. Is this something aid agencies should do in large camps for displaced people in isolated rural areas such as Darfur?*

This service requires both expertise and a longer-term commitment. If people are made aware of their status then there must be a mechanism in place to provide other services such as provision of antiretrovirals. If an aid agency sees the importance of such a service but does not have the relevant skills, it should lobby for a service to be provided.

5. *Is the training of TBAs (traditional birth attendants) to carry out AIDS-awareness and to prevent infection a good way to mainstream?*

   Where TBAs are already working in the community and are respected sources of information, they may be good intermediaries for disseminating culturally appropriate information on HIV transmission.

6. *Does HIV affect malaria rates and should we give insecticide-treated nets to all HIV-positive persons?*

   HIV infection does increase both the incidence and severity of malaria.[38] The effect of malaria on HIV is still being researched but it is thought that malaria does increase the viral load in the body – this means that the person may progress faster to the AIDS stage and the transmission of HIV is increased. Malaria is also more frequent and severe in HIV-positive pregnant women. It is difficult to know who is HIV-positive and as net supply is often limited, it is difficult to cover all potentially infected persons. In high-prevalence countries you may consider giving more nets to each family and encouraging families to sleep close to nets in order to take advantage of the halo effect.[39]

7. *How can we mainstream in a way that is culturally appropriate in countries where sex is rarely discussed?*

   It is always good to look to the national staff for direction. The Ministry of Health usually has a national AIDS control programme that may or may not have produced material for informing people about HIV and AIDS. Religious considerations also need to be taken into account – again the national staff can assist. Discussing chronic illness and sexually transmitted diseases in general is often a good starting point.

8. *As a manager, do I need to consider having PEP available for women who have been sexually assaulted?*

   Yes, you should make yourself aware of agencies in the area that can provide this facility. Remember that it has to be taken within 72 hours and the treatment is a month-long course which should be medically supervised. Psycho-social counselling, pregnancy testing, and treatment for STIs is normally also offered. In Uganda, all emergency 'quick run bags'[40] contain PEP; in other programmes there is an agreement with Médecins Sans Frontières.

9. *Will mainstreaming HIV and AIDS mean more work for the staff?*

It is more a case of thinking differently than having additional activities; as with both gender and accountability, mainstreaming HIV and AIDS should be considered as another element of good programme practice. There will however be some additional work such as training and awarenes-raising for national staff, national organisation partners, and people in the community. This manual is designed to help managers address these issues so that mainstreaming does not become just another 'add-on.'

10. *Why are HIV-positive people different from other vulnerable groups such as those with a chronic illness?*

They are not. In most emergencies it is not possible to know who is HIV-positive and who is not. We usually target those households where someone is chronically ill so as not to discriminate against HIV-positive people. The only difference is that HIV-positive people can transmit the virus and need to know how to prevent transmission.

11. *People are reluctant to say they are HIV-positive – how can we know?*

You cannot know. As above, treat people who are chronically ill as potentially HIV-positive, but do not discriminate. Remember, many HIV-positive people are healthy and able to function normally. There could easily be staff members who are HIV-positive and they have the right of confidentiality regarding their status.

Section 5:
Activities and exercises

This section contains 12 activities which can be used in various combinations in the following situations:

- Induction of new staff
- A one-day training for staff
- Community meetings for gathering and sharing information
- A one-day training for community members including hygiene promoters, pump attendants, and other project volunteers

First we will outline these different situations and then we will present the 12 activities in detail. See Appendix 4 for cards to use in some of these activities.

5.1 Induction for staff

Mainstreaming HIV and AIDS should be both internal (workplace) and external (programmes and partners). Accordingly all staff should have some basic knowledge of HIV and of the process of mainstreaming. In order to be able to talk about HIV and other intimate subjects, staff need to be clear about how they feel: what are their beliefs, values, assumptions, and attitudes?

In an emergency, inductions are often brief and cover the minimum amount of information. On HIV mainstreaming the minimum would be:

- Check that the person knows all the basic facts, especially about prevention and the risk of HIV transmission for themselves and the community (see Appendix 1)
- Ensure that condoms are available and staff know how to access them if they choose to

- Make sure that the workplace policy is available even if there is no time to go through it
- Explain and get the staff member to sign the Code of Conduct[41]
- Give the person the name/s of people who can be contacted in the field for more information and/or condoms

5.2 A one-day training for staff

Objectives

- To ensure that staff understand the concept of mainstreaming in programming
- To ensure that staff understand the concept of mainstreaming and how it is practised in the particular programme
- To ensure that staff understand their roles and responsibilities in mainstreaming

Time	Activity	Subject	Resources needed
9.00–9.30	1	Introductions, objectives, and knowledge test	Paper, pens
9.30–10.00	3	Values clarification	Large pieces of paper
	4	The beans game	Beans – two colours
10.00–10.30		Tea	
10.30–11.30	5	Looking at how the emergency has affected/ been affected by HIV and AIDS	Flip charts and pens
11.30–12.30		Questions and discussions	
12.30–13.30		Lunch	
13.30–14.30	7	Case study	Flip chart paper and pens
14.30–15.00	8	Planning for action	
15.30–16.00		Tea	
16.00–17.00	12	Voting for focal points Evaluation of course	Evaluation forms, post-its or flip chart paper

5.3 Community meetings

Objectives

- To explore the basic knowledge of HIV and AIDS in the community and to correct inaccurate beliefs
- To map out how the community has been affected by HIV and AIDS
- To plan collectively how to mainstream HIV and AIDS

Time

It is always difficult to judge how long community meetings take, as people seldom arrive on time and there are formal presentations and speeches that need to be factored in to the programme. On average, meetings should not last longer than about an hour before taking a break.

Activities for community meetings

All of the activities listed below can be carried out with the community. However, bearing in mind the time constraints above, you should not plan to do too many activities on one day. You could do two activities and then plan another session on another day; community people have other tasks even if they are in a refugee or IDP camp.

- Activity 2 – basic knowledge using three pile sorting
- Activity 5 – how the emergency has affected/been affected by HIV and AIDS
- Activity 9 – mapping of affected and infected
- Activity 10 – planning
- Activity 11 – recognising stigma

Preparing to talk to communities about HIV

Discussions about HIV and AIDS and sexual matters with communities can be difficult, and not everyone feels comfortable leading these discussions. It is best to select someone who knows the community, can speak the language, and who feels comfortable talking about sexual matters with community members. Use partner organisations if possible, especially if they have been working in the communities before the emergency.

Introduce the subject through the public health promotion activities and ask permission first to talk about HIV. It could be that a focus group is held with different groups: women, leaders, and if possible teenagers first. This will be a chance to gauge the level of understanding and the degree of openness on the subject. It may be that you have to talk about general health issues first and then gradually introduce the subject. Follow the advice of local staff and key community leaders.

Some other points to consider are:

- Avoid moralising and preaching. Give facts and let people make their own decisions – even if your religion does not condone condoms you cannot allow this to influence your discussion. If you are totally against condoms, ask someone else to do the HIV prevention work.

- Build on what the community already knows and use culturally appropriate examples.

- Encourage support for those who are affected and possibly infected.

- If there is anyone who has been brave enough to 'come out' about their HIV status, you could use him or her for discussions with community members – but do not ask for volunteers to do this. HIV-positive people need to take the initiative to come forward by themselves. There may be a local NGO where members are open about their status and happy to talk to others about it.

- Know when to stop – if the discussion becomes too embarrassing or accusing, stop.

5.4 A one-day training for community members

This session is for hygiene promoters, pump attendants, and other project volunteers.

Objectives

- To ensure that everyone is aware of the facts about HIV and AIDS transmission and prevention
- To explore the issue of stigma and how to deal with it
- To look at how the current emergency situation is affected by/is affecting the AIDS epidemic
- To plan an appropriate community response

Time	Activity	Subject	Resources needed
9.00–9.30	4	Introduction Beans game	Beans in two colours
9.30–10.30	2	Three pile sorting on knowledge	Coloured pictures on small cards
10.30–11.30		Tea	
11.30–12.30	11	Recognising stigma	Flip chart paper and pens
12.30–13.30		Lunch	
13.30–14.30	5	How HIV affects emergencies How emergencies affect HIV rates	Flip chart paper and pens
14.30–15.30	8 – external part of exercise	Sector response	Flip chart paper and pens
15.30–16.00		Tea	
16.00–16.30		Plenary	
16.30–17.00	12	Evaluation	Small pieces of paper with smiling/non-smiling faces (one on each side)

5.5 Activities

Activity 1: Knowledge test

Objective: to test people's knowledge of HIV and AIDS

Time: ten minutes, plus ten minutes' discussion

Target audience: project staff

Tools: printouts of questions

Get everyone to complete the following test and go through the answers with each person. It is important that there are no gaps in knowledge or misconceptions. The answers should be 'Agree' to all except number five.

1	AIDS stands for Acquired Immunodeficiency Syndrome	Agree/Disagree
2	There are four ways of transmission: • Sexual • Mother to baby • Blood products • Exchange of infected blood through needles, razor blades, and other piercing instruments	Agree/Disagree
3	Without treatment, AIDS is fatal	Agree/Disagree
4	You cannot get infected through: • Kissing • Eating together • Hugging • Sharing clothes	Agree/Disagree
5	People have been cured by traditional medicines	Agree/Disagree
6	If you start on antiretrovirals, you have to do it for life	Agree/Disagree

Activity 2: Basic knowledge using three pile sorting

Objective: to test out local knowledge

Target audience: community members and volunteers

Time: anything up to an hour

Tools: picture cards

This is best done as a discussion in groups divided according to gender. Ask about beliefs in the community and also find out the local names for parts of the body in order to be able to use these whilst talking to the community. If there is a local NGO working in the area, ask them to join you and to help lead the discussion.

You can photocopy the cards depicting ways of transmission, ways of not getting HIV, and prevention (Appendix 4). Make two or three copies of each card. Muddle these up and give a pile to each group. Get people to sort them into piles: ways of transmission, ways you cannot get HIV and AIDS, and prevention methods. Then have a discussion especially about traditional beliefs or misconceptions.

You can also pick out some cards at random and ask people to explain to the whole group why it is or is not a method of transmission. Do the same with prevention cards.

Activity 3: Values clarification

Objective: to challenge some of the misconceptions and beliefs that people may have

Target audience: project staff

Time: 30 minutes

Tools: two pieces of A4 paper, one headed 'Agree' and the other 'Disagree', and some tape

The suggested statements opposite are deliberately provocative in order to stimulate discussion and to get people to think about their views. You can also present the positive version of each of these statements, but experience has shown that this is not nearly as productive for a good discussion.

Put up two signs at opposite ends of the room – one 'Agree' and one 'Disagree'. Everyone stands in the middle of the room whilst the facilitator reads out a statement. People should then move quickly to either one or other of the signs – they should not take any time to consider their reply. Photos can be taken of the groups and repeated after the training in order to see if people have changed their views. After each statement, have a quick discussion with the group.

Some suggested statements (choose three or four of these):

People who are HIV-positive have been irresponsible – it is their own fault

HIV and AIDS can be prevented and nobody should become infected

If you do not know your HIV status you do not need to protect yourself

Only immoral people contract HIV

If I were HIV-positive, I would hide the fact from my family

Women are flirtatious and cause men to have multiple partners

People who carry condoms are promiscuous

HIV testing should be compulsory

Using condoms takes all the pleasure out of sex

In an emergency we should prioritise those who are HIV-negative

Some suggested points to bring up in a discussion:

Not judging others against our own religious or moral standards

Being too quick to judge others before you know the whole story

Not looking at the circumstances that may lead people to behave in a risky manner

Not having enough information about something (for example condom use)

Being comfortable with talking about sensitive issues with people

Considering that if someone has strong opinions about something, they may not be the right person to train or to talk to communities

Activity 4: The beans game

Objective: to show how quickly the virus can be spread. It is also good as an icebreaker as it requires some movement and interaction and gets everyone thinking about the way the virus could spread.

Target audience: project staff and volunteers

Time: 30 minutes including discussion

Tools: a bag of beans where there are two distinct colours – say red and white

Divide the beans into two piles – the red ones should represent the known prevalence of HIV in the relevant country – say 10 per cent of the whole. Give everyone three beans but make sure 10 per cent of the group receive red beans and everyone else white beans.

Get everyone to wander around talking to as many people as possible. Every time they meet someone new, they should exchange a bean. After about ten minutes, get everyone to stand in a circle and show their beans to the rest of the group. Everyone should now have a mixture of red and white beans. Explain that the red beans are the virus (after asking if anyone can guess what they represent) and make sure everyone understands the point of the exercise.

Activity 5: Looking at how the emergency has affected/been affected by HIV and AIDS

Objective: to explore how the emergency has affected/been affected by the epidemic

Target audience: staff and community volunteers

Time: one hour

Tools: flip chart paper, pens, and tape

You can split the group into smaller groups and get people to brainstorm on how HIV affects the emergency and how the emergency affects the HIV situation. Use the examples in Section 2 and Appendix 2 to get people thinking about their particular country. Write these on flip charts and discuss them together.

Activity 6: How HIV and AIDS can or has affected our community

Objective: to find out how the community has been affected by the epidemic

Target audience: community members

Time: anything up to an hour

Tools: flip chart paper, pens, and tape, if people can read and write

In separate groups, ask for suggestions as to how the HIV and AIDS epidemic has affected or could affect the lives of the people in the community. If people are reluctant to talk about AIDS it may be better to start with discussing chronic illness and STIs. This could be done during the emergency but also during the recovery phase. The example opposite shows some of the suggestions from a community in East Africa.

Example: How HIV and AIDS has affected our community

People

More people falling ill or dying

More young people and workers falling ill

More children having to cope alone

More children having to look after other children and having to
work to make money

It's hard coping with so much death

Old people have no one to pass on community knowledge to

We have to spend time looking after the sick rather than
working in the fields

Money matters

Sick people cost money

Carers' incomes are decreased or are lost

Funerals are expensive

We need to hire help in the fields when people are sick

Sometimes we sell our assets to buy medicine

Food and livelihoods

We can't grow as much food as there are fewer people to work
in the fields

We have fewer animals, as we have had to sell some
to buy medicines

It is expensive to buy food and sometimes money is short

The doctor says our sick people need good food
but it is expensive

If someone is weak, it is difficult to plough
or to herd the goats

Activity 7: Case study

Objective: to explore what action the different sectors would take to mainstream HIV and AIDS in an emergency

Target audience: project staff

Time: one hour with discussion

Tools: print outs of case study, flip chart paper, pens, and tape

Go through the case study and make sure everyone understands. Divide people into groups and ask them to answer the questions. You may want to divide the groups into managers, human resources staff, public health staff, and livelihoods staff, depending on how many staff you have in the group.

Discuss the answers together and then compare with the possible answers in Appendix 3.

Case study

The people from country X have fled across the border to country Z and have settled around the town of Y. This town is on the main trucking route and is a business centre, especially during the tobacco auction time in August and September. Although prostitution is illegal in country Z, there are known to be commercial sex workers at truck stops, bars, and other places of entertainment.

The refugees are mostly from a Muslim pastoral community and have walked about 40 kilometres to get to this town. There are many women-headed households as the men have stayed on to fight in the civil war.

It has been decided to do water, sanitation, and hygiene promotion in the camps that have been set up, and also to assist other agencies with food distribution before moving into livelihoods work.

- What background information would you require on HIV and AIDS during your rapid assessment?
- From where might you get this?
- Human resources staff – you employ new national staff and have planned a one-day induction for them. What would you include for HIV mainstreaming?
- Food security and livelihoods staff – what could you do on HIV mainstreaming in the first month?
- Public health promotion and water and sanitation staff – what might you want to consider during the start-up of your programme?
- Managers – what measures might you suggest during co-ordination meetings for good IDP/refugee camp management to reduce the risk of HIV transmission?

Activity 8: Planning for action in the programme

External

Objective: to plan how to mainstream HIV and AIDS externally

Target audience: project staff and volunteers

Time: 30 minutes with discussion

Tools: flip chart paper, pens, and tape

Discuss as a group and write a work plan that is appropriate and feasible given the limits of the situation. The work plan could look something like this:

When	What	Who
Assessment	Use Section 3 (page 21)	Assessment team staff
Implementation	Use suggestions in section 3 (page 27)	Technical team
Staff recruitment and induction	• Make sure everyone is aware of Code of Conduct and workplace policy • Mainstreaming training • Condoms made available	Human resources staff Recruiting managers
Monitoring	• Are the measures we put in place working? • Have the staff and beneficiaries received the knowledge and resources they need to prevent infection and to mitigate effects of the epidemic and the emergency?	Technical staff Human resources staff Monitoring and evaluation officer
Evaluation	How successful was the mainstreaming in the emergency?	Evaluation team

Internal

Objective: to come up with plans for internal mainstreaming

Target audience: project staff

Time: 30 minutes

Tools: flip chart paper, pens, and tape

There are several ways you can mainstream in the workplace:

- Make sure everyone is aware of the workplace policy, the gender policy, and the Code of Conduct
- Discuss whether staff would like a focal point – a person in the office to whom they can go for information and assistance
- Hold training sessions for staff

Activity 9: Mapping of affected and infected

Objective: to find out how many vulnerable households there are in the community

Target audience: community members

Time: anything up to an hour

Tools: flip chart paper and pens or sticks, stones, and other materials for drawing on the ground

Decide with the community how you will define a vulnerable household (this is not intended to be only HIV-affected households but all vulnerable households where there are chronically ill people, orphans (OVCs), or female-headed or child-headed households. Look at how many carers there are for the chronically ill people in one household (for example if there is one carer and three people who are ill, there is a high caring burden). There may be a local NGO which has already identified households and therefore could assist with the exercise.

If it is feasible and acceptable, draw an actual map of the community and mark in the vulnerable households. Ask:

- What will these households need in the way of extra help?
- How could this be provided (by Oxfam, others, the community)?
- What do we need in the way of extra resources including training?
- Where should we place facilities such as latrines and water points in order to make it easier for these households?

Activity 10: Planning

Objective: to plan mainstreaming at community level

Target audience: community members

Time: up to an hour

Tools: none

After Activity 9, the community needs to make a plan of what to do, how to do it, and who will do it. Remember that it will probably include other local NGO partners, and make sure that staff do not promise anything that is more than the programme has planned to do. It is better to be honest and try and find a local partner who can assist.

Activity 11: Recognising stigma[42]

Objective: to explore the issues of stigma and how to overcome it

Target audience: community members and volunteers

Time: one hour

Tools: flip chart paper and pens

Ask participants to draw three circles, starting with an inner circle, followed by a middle circle, and then an outer circle. Then ask the participants to identify someone from their family, preferably someone who is with them in their present place of living. Draw this person as a stick figure in the inner circle. Next, the participants should imagine someone in the community, a neighbour or friend who is placed in the middle circle. In the outer circle, participants should put someone who is from outside the community – a famous person or one of the aid agency staff.

Ask participants to close their eyes and to visualise all these people they have identified. They should then try to imagine that all these people are HIV-positive.

Ask for volunteers to discuss what came into their minds when they were thinking about the different people, especially those in the inner and middle circles. Ask them to consider:

- How do you feel about the risk of you becoming infected from these people?
- Would your behaviour towards them change in any way?
- How would the knowledge of their condition change your way of interacting with them?
- Is there a difference in the way you think of them in the inner, middle, and outer circle?

Now ask the volunteers to draw themselves in the inner circle and get them to imagine that they are also HIV-positive. Ask them to consider:

- How does it feel?
- What would you want people to do for you especially now in the emergency?
- Would it make any difference to the life you have now or the one you had before the emergency?

Getting people to role-play stigma is also a good discussion point. One way of doing a role-play is to use a method called 'Story with a Gap' – where the role-play depicts a certain scenario but the actors stop before a solution is found and they invite members of the audience to come up and complete the play.

Activity 12: Evaluation of the course

Objective: to evaluate the course

Target audience: all course participants – both staff and volunteers

Time: 20 minutes

Tools: paper and pens

There are several ways to do this:

- Formal evaluation using a short questionnaire
- Getting people to put smiling/non-smiling faces next to pre-determined questions on flip charts
- Group evaluations where everyone has to come to a consensus
- The fun ball game:
    - Give everyone a piece of paper, which has on one side a smiling face and on the other an unhappy face
    - Get everyone to write a useful thing they learnt and something that was not so useful under the two faces
    - Take the pages and scrunch them up so that they form a ball with layers of paper
    - Get everyone to stand in a circle
    - Throw the ball to one person who peels off a piece of paper and reads out both the useful and not so useful things people have learnt
    - The person throws the ball to someone else who also peels off a paper and reads out the comments
    - Continue round the circle until all the comments have been read out

Keep the comments to help you when you are planning the next training session.

Section 6:
Summary

Stembile's Summary of Important Points to Remember

- Remember that mainstreaming is keeping the focus of your humanitarian programme but thinking about how not to worsen the HIV epidemic, and making sure that you consider the needs of those who are affected or infected
- Avoid stigmatisation – use vulnerable households or chronically ill as criteria
- If possible find out as much as you can about the HIV and AIDS situation in your country before the emergency
- Remember that there must always be a minimum response
- Assess the risks situation by using the scoring system (page 24)
- In water and sanitation consider the safety and protection of vulnerable groups as well as convenience and accessibility of services
- Consider cultural and religious issues in education and always take advice from local staff and communities
- Do not allow your own prejudices or religious views to guide the response
- Make sure your staff are well informed about HIV facts, services available, what they can expect of their employer, and what is expected of them
- Breast is best in emergencies for the first four to six months, with a short weaning period
- Think about improved nutrition for HIV-positive people
- Livelihoods should be suited to the special needs of both those infected and affected
- Consider gender, accountability, and protection as part of good programming

Appendix 1:
Everything you may have forgotten about HIV and AIDS[43]

What is HIV?

HIV stands for human immunodeficiency virus. If you have the virus in your body you are HIV-positive.

What is AIDS?

AIDS stands for acquired immunodeficiency syndrome. After some time, HIV damages the immune system so that the person becomes vulnerable to a group of illnesses and infections (called opportunistic infections). The immune system of a person without HIV would normally be able to fight off these infections. If one or more opportunistic infections are found in a person with HIV, that person is said to have AIDS.

Where does it come from?

No one knows for sure where the virus comes from, although it has been around in Africa for about 30 years. The latest thinking is that the virus mutated from one affecting animals to one affecting humans. This occurred through the contact of humans with chimpanzee blood during the killing of these animals for food.

Does everyone who is HIV-positive get AIDS?

If people who are HIV-positive do not take antiretroviral drugs, they will get AIDS. The time it takes to move from one state to the other varies according to the type of virus, the person's nutritional status and their access to health care. Once infected, the person will always carry the virus in their blood and can infect others.

How is the virus spread?

There are only four ways that the virus can be spread:

- Through unprotected sexual intercourse (where no condom is used), whether homosexual or heterosexual
- Through getting infected blood into your bloodstream (by infected blood transfusions)
- From contaminated needles, syringes, and other piercing equipment
- From an infected mother to her baby before and during birth or by breast-feeding

Ways in which it is not spread

- Everyday contact at work, school, or home
- Kissing, hugging, touching, and handshakes
- Sharing food or utensils
- Eating from the same dish
- Sharing telephones
- Toilet seats
- Public baths or swimming pools
- Mosquito or other insect bites
- The communion cup in Christian churches

Can you tell if someone is HIV-positive?

It may take several years for HIV to damage the immune system so much that a person becomes ill. During these years a person with HIV may look and feel well; they may not even know they have the virus. The person is infected with HIV but does not have AIDS. The only way of proving that someone is HIV-positive is by blood tests after the window period.

What is the window period?

The virus is detectable in the blood (through testing) two to three weeks after the person has been infected. Sometimes it takes longer but the majority of people can be tested positive within three months of exposure. This time between being infected and the virus showing up in the blood is known as the window period.

How can the spread of the virus be prevented?

- Safer sex – using a condom or non-penetrative sex
- Making sure all blood transfusions are tested and discarded if found to be HIV-positive
- Using disposable needles and syringes for injections
- Using a new razor blade each time for cutting the umbilical cord, scarification, tattooing, or in public barber shops
- Exclusively breast-feeding for the first three to six months, with a short weaning period
- Giving a pregnant woman antiretroviral treatment specifically to prevent mother-to-child transmission

Is there a cure for HIV and AIDS?

There is no medication at present that will remove the virus from the blood of an infected person. Antiretroviral drugs slow the transition from HIV-positive to full-blown AIDS but they do not stop the person from being able to infect others. Traditional medicine, magic, or prayers have so far not proved to be effective in removing the virus from the bloodstream of HIV-positive people. There is currently no vaccine available against the virus.

Appendix 2:
Factors increasing HIV in emergencies, and possible responses

Level	Factors	Responses
Macro environment	Political and economic discrimination Poverty/health care Political instability War/conflict	Creating an organisational strategy including an HIV workplace policy inclusive of non-discrimination, policy for illness, and the right to confidentiality. Training staff in stigmatisation. Creating and enforcing a Code of Conduct. Organisational campaigns: having access to services for all, lowering costs of treatment and setting up a mechanism for staff to access this information. Finding out if there are laws in the country to protect people with HIV. Creating relations with the govern-ment (if there is one in place) and advocating for change in laws and policies if necessary. Using a human rights-based approach to programming: applying protection principles and basic rights information dissemination. Collaborating with other organisations in the creation of reporting mechanisms for violence and crime.

Level	Factors	Responses
Emergency environment	Gender inequity	Using gender-sensitive programming
	Sexual and gender-based violence	Mainstreaming protection issues in programming: involving women in decisions about site and shelter planning
	Lack of protection	
	Overcrowding	
	Security of latrines, facilities, fuel, food, water	Including chronically ill people in a vulnerability assessment (no need for HIV and AIDS as separate criteria)
	Rape and HIV as weapons of war	
	Survival/transactional sex; commercial sex	Using an integrated multi-sectoral approach via partners or networking with other agencies
	Demobilisation	
	Lack of support for PLWHA	Carrying out income generation activities, targeting women and youth
	Presence of military	
	Peacekeeping	
	Lack of health infrastructure, leading to non-availability of: sexual health services, screened blood, sterile equipment, voluntary counselling and testing, TB control, care for PLWHA, mother-to-child transmission prevention services	Using a livelihoods approach for food insecurity, such as cash for work
		Involving youth in project planning and design; vocational training
		Involving PLWHA in project planning and design (NB this depends on contextual environment – are there existing support groups?)
	Increased exposure of PLWHA to other sicknesses (especially TB, diarrhoeal diseases, and malaria)	Highlighting and fighting stigma where possible
	Mixing of host and displaced populations	Targeting health promotion activities at military
	Decrease of labour pool in areas of high prevalence	Supporting treatment and care services through partner organisations
		Doing public health promotion and public health engineering to promote and maintain health and decrease water-related diseases (targeting areas of high HIV prevalence)

Level	Factors	Responses
		Doing malaria control programmes
		Targeting youth and transitional areas for demo-bilisation with public health promotion
		Training in life skills for women and youth, and condom negotiation skills (also involving men)
		Focusing on individuals; careful targeting; protection (no forced repatriation, confidentiality, non-discrimi-nation)
		Ensuring that host and displaced populations are involved in programme planning and design
		Ensuring mitigation of impacts by labour sharing, labour saving devices, and divisible assets
Behavioural	Psychological impacts: wish to repopulate; fatalism	Public health promotion with safe sex messages including provision of condoms (targeting youth and transitional areas for demo-bilisation)
	Multiple sexual partners	
	Boredom/alcohol/drug use	
	Lack of condom use	
	Lack of knowledge of HIV and AIDS; myths and incorrect information	Promoting WHO guidelines for those handling blood and body fluids
	Unwanted pregnancy	Doing vocational training (involving youth and alterna-tive activities targeting men)
	Mother-to-child transmission	
	Pregnancy at an early age	Supporting treatment and care services through partner organisations (STI treatment, TB control, voluntary counselling and testing, home-based care, mother-to-child transmission prevention services, etc.)

Level	Factors	Responses
		Promoting safe infant feeding
		Challenging social norms (schooling, employment, inheritance laws)
		Challenging norms that allow/encourage men to have multiple sexual partners
Biomedical	Virus subtypes	Supporting treatment and care services through partner organisations (STI treatment, TB control, voluntary counselling and testing, home-based care, mother-to-child transmission prevention services, etc.)
	Stage of infection	
	Presence of other STIs	
	Male circumcision (protective[44])	
	Female genital mutilation	
	Physiology (females are more susceptible)	Incorporating cultural information into programmes

Appendix 3:
Suggestions for answers to Activity 7 (Case study)

Background information

Look at pages 19 to 47 in Section 3.

Sources: UNAIDS website, Ministry of Health, UNAIDS office, WHO office, other NGOs, local HIV and AIDS resource centre, health staff and clinic records if available. VCT centre data may be confidential and staff may be reluctant to give it out.

Human resources staff

- General knowledge about HIV – transmission, prevention, and treatment
- Code of Conduct
- Workplace policy
- General discussion on cultural and religious concerns
- Tell them who the focal point in the office is and what they can expect from this person
- In a high-prevalence country, you may need to consider what to do if your staff fall sick – maybe hire extra numbers to compensate

Food security and livelihoods

- Make sure drivers are given information and have access to condoms
- Make sure there is no chance for coercion among those distributing food or non-food items
- Find out who are the vulnerable households who may require extra rations
- Encourage breast-feeding

- Plan for livelihoods that are appropriate for carers with little time or people weakened by the virus

Public health promotion and water and sanitation staff

- Consider convenient latrines and water points for vulnerable households
- Discuss needs with identified vulnerable households
- Consider special hygiene kits for vulnerable households
- Plan for later HIV information mainstreaming in the community

Managers

- Lobby for safe facilities such as well-lit latrines and water points that women can use without harassment
- Lobby for services such as VCT, PEP, and antiretrovirals
- Have a system in place for whistle blowing for inappropriate behaviour by staff or national/international troops

Appendix 4: Activity cards

You can photocopy these cards, colour and laminate them, and use them in different activities such as three pile sorting (Activity 2). They represent non-transmission routes, transmission routes, and prevention.

Non-transmission routes

1 eating together
2 arms round one another
3 a latrine
4 using a mobile phone
5 hugging
6 swimming together
7 mosquito
8 bedbug and tick
9 woman selling second hand clothes
10 toothbrush

Transmission routes

11 couple having sex
12 blood transfusion
13 getting a tattoo
14 ear piercing
15 getting an injection from a non-medical person
16 woman having a baby
17 breast-feeding

Prevention

18 condom
19 saying no to girl friends
20 husband and wife
21 new razor blade
22 clean syringe used by a medical person
23 traditional healer
24 pills

Card 1

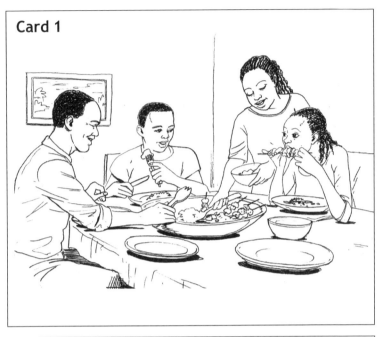

Card 2

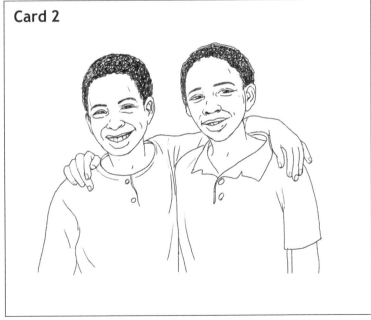

Card 3

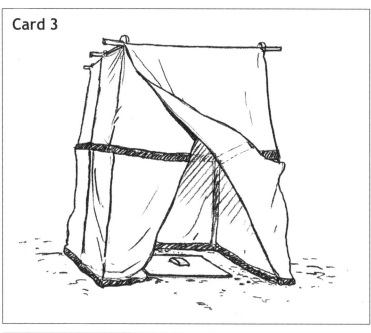

Card 4

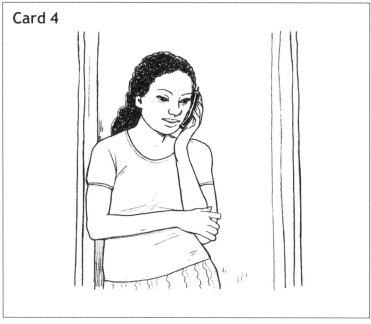

Card 5

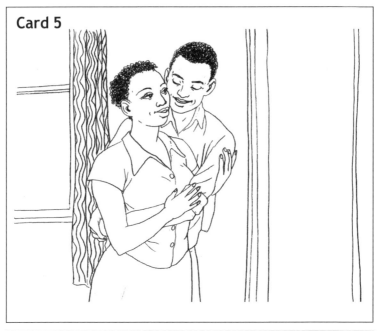

Card 6

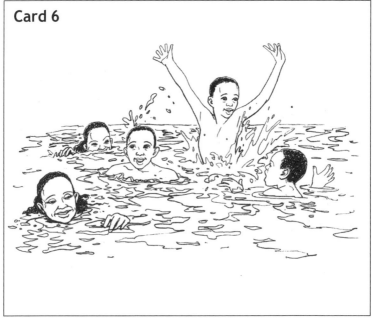

Card 7

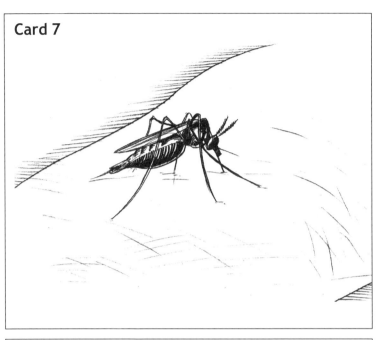

Card 8

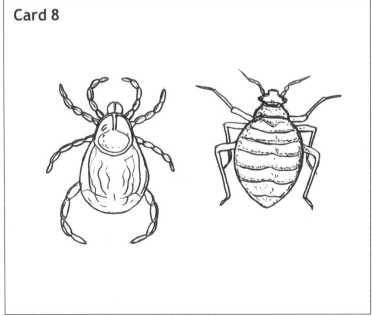

Card 9

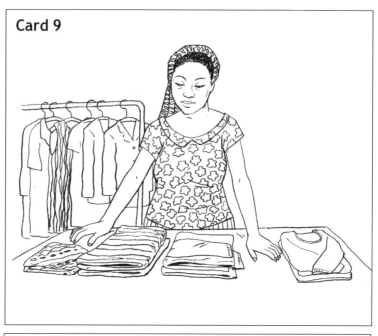

Card 10

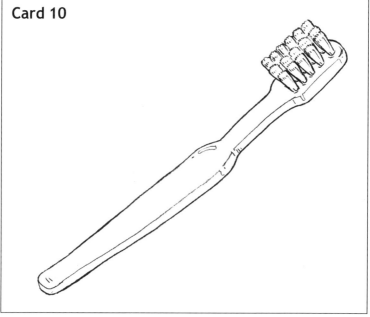

Card 11

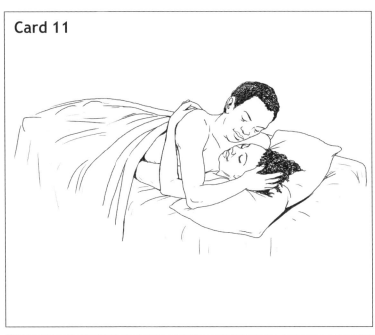

Card 12

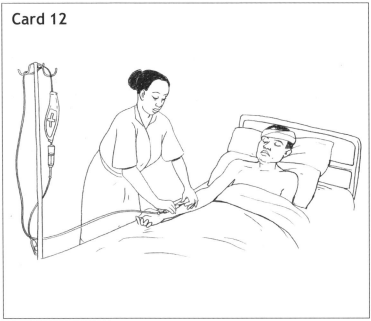

Card 13

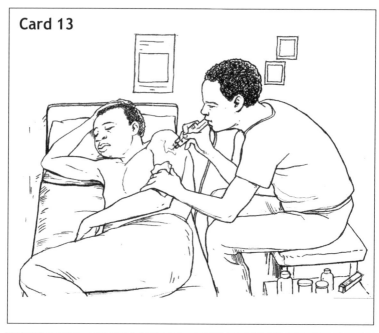

Card 14

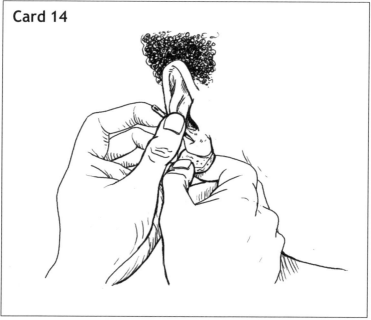

Card 15

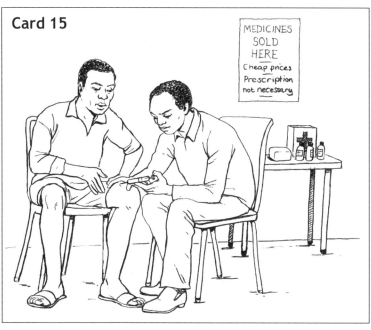

Card 16

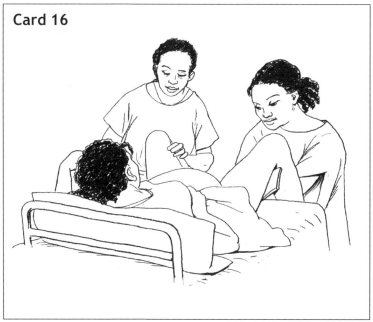

Card 17

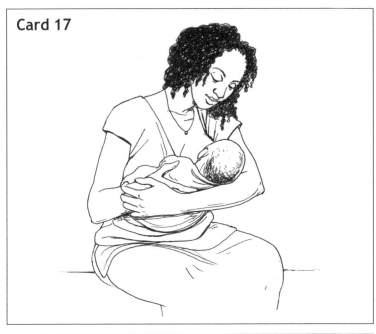

Card 18

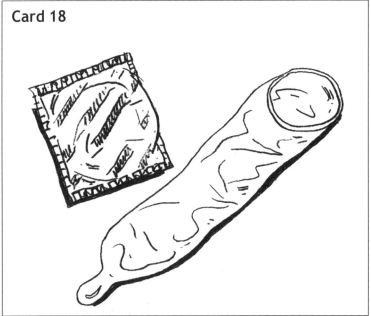

Card 19

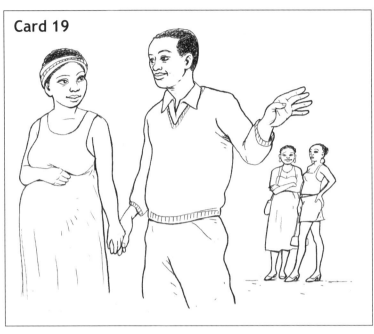

Card 20

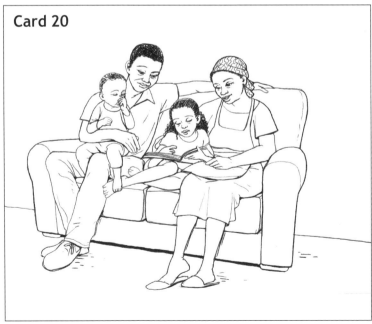

Card 21

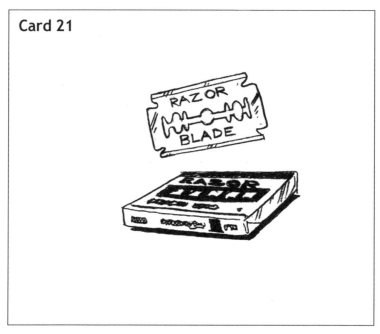

Card 22

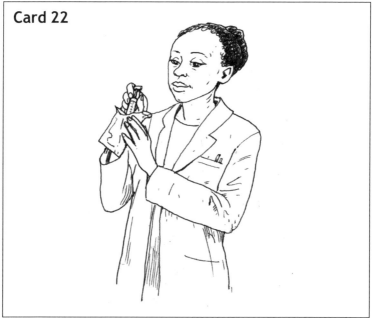

Card 23

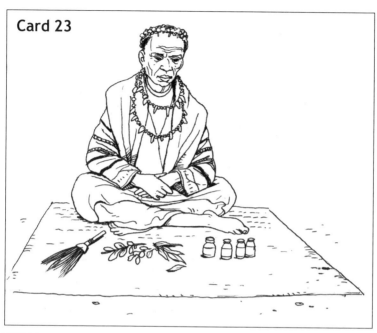

Card 24

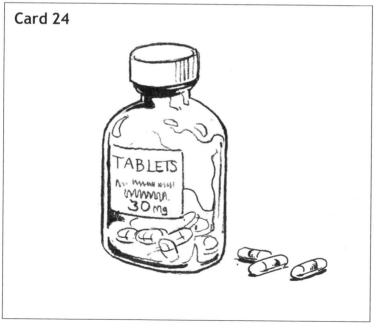

Notes

1   S. Maddock (2002) 'Making modernisation work: new narratives, change strategies and people management in the public sector', *International Journal of Public Sector Management* 15 (1): 13–43.

2   The Sphere Project (2004).

3   Gender must be considered because transmission from men to women is more common, and protection must be considered because in an emergency rape or selling sexual favours for survival often occur, increasing the chances of HIV transmission.

4   Opportunistic infections occur because a person's immune system is so weak that it cannot fight off unusual infections.

5   By 'chronically ill people', we mean all those with a long-term illness that may or may not include those who are weakened by the virus and suffer from chronic conditions such as debilitating diarrhoea or intermittent fevers.

6   Angola and Sierre Leone are two examples – see P. B. Spiegel (2004) 'HIV/AIDS among conflict-affected and displaced populations: dispelling myths and taking action', *Disasters* 28 (3): 322–39.

7   See Amnesty International 'Women and war', http://web.amnesty.org/actforwomen/conflict-2-eng (accessed October 2006).

8   Documented recently in West Africa by Save the Children UK, http://news.bbc.co.uk/2/hi/africa/4983378.stm (accessed October 2006).

9   A.J. Khaw, P. Salama, B. Burkholder, and T.J. Dondero (2000) 'HIV risk and prevention in emergency-affected populations: a review', *Disasters* 24 (3): 181–97.

10 There is evidence to suggest that the use of alcohol can be associated with high-risk sexual behaviours. See http://pubs.niaaa.nih.gov/publications/aa57.htm (accessed October 2006).

11 UNAIDS (2004) 'Report on the Global AIDS Epidemic, AIDS and conflict: a growing problem worldwide', http://www.unaids.org/bangkok2004/GAR2004_html/GAR2004_00_en.htm.

12 N. Mock (2004) 'Conflict and HIV: a framework for risk assessment to prevent HIV in conflict-affected settings in Africa', *Emerging Themes in Epidemiology* 1 (6).

13 V.M. Walden, K. Mwangulube and P. Makhumula-Nkhoma (1999) 'Measuring the impact of a behaviour change intervention for commercial sex workers and their potential clients', *Malawi Health Education Research* 14 (4): 545–54.

14 At least half of today's 15-year-olds in sub-Saharan Africa are likely to contract HIV at some point in their lifetime. In Botswana a 15-year-old boy has a 95 per cent risk of contracting HIV in his lifetime.

15 Men who have sex with men (MSM) are a marginalised minority in many developing countries where homosexuality may be either illegal or socially unacceptable. Some 82 developing countries have laws against MSM, making this a hard to reach group for any prevention project, and even more so in emergency programmes.

16 Here, by health care we mean drugs (including antiretrovirals) and safe blood transfusions.

17 Post exposure prophylaxis is an antiretroviral treatment given immediately after exposure to the virus (for example after unprotected sex) to prevent the person from becoming HIV-positive.

18 http://www.ifrc.org/PUBLICAT/conduct/code.asp.

19 This would give you an idea of opportunistic infections among 15–45 year olds – the group most likely to be HIV-positive.

20 See S. Ferron et al. (2002).

21 It is difficult to talk openly about HIV and AIDS when there is little buy-in from the host government.

22 Adapted from FHI/PATH (2002).

23 See P. Creti and S. Jaspars (2006) *Cash transfer programming in emergencies; a practical guide*, Oxford: Oxfam.

24 For adults and adolescents, during the asymptomatic phase energy requirements increase by 10 per cent, and during the symptomatic phase energy requirements increase by 20 to 30 per cent. For children, during the asymptomatic phase energy requirements increase by 10 per cent. In the symptomatic phase with no weight loss a 20 per cent increase in energy is required, whilst in the symptomatic phase *with* weight loss an increase of 50 to 100 per cent is needed.

25 This area is currently being studied. See W.W. Fawzi et al (2004).

26 A weak immune system increases the risk for opportunistic infections for PLWHA.

27 Four to six months being the age when infants are able to eat solids and tolerate cows' milk.

28 P. J. Iliff, E. G. Piwoz, N. V. Tavengwa et al. (2005) 'Early exclusive breastfeeding reduces the risk of postnatal HIV-1 transmission and increases HIV-free survival', *AIDS* 19 (7): 699–708.

29   WHO/UNFPA/UNICEF/UNAIDS (2004) 'HIV transmission through breastfeeding: a review of available evidence', WHO.

30   Using the chronically ill criteria as well as OVCs and child-headed households.

31   Supplementing the ration with Corn Soya Blend (CSB) where the general food distribution is inadequate could result in the CSB being distributed too widely within the household or sold on the market for cash income.

32   J. Cabassi (2004) *Renewing our voice: Code of good practice for NGOs responding to HIV/AIDS*, Geneva: The NGO HIV/AIDS Code of Practice Project, http://www.aidsalliance.org/sw21331.asp.

33   A proxy indicator is one that is used to measure something for which no direct information is available, either because it would be too expensive or may be unreliable. An example of this is an indicator for malaria rate reduction which could be the number of people sleeping under an insecticide-treated net every night.

34   Indicators to measure the process, how things are going and the outputs of an activity.

35   Indicators to measure the impact of the project and the outcome of an activity.

36   http://www.ennonline.net/ife/report/Monitoring.html.

37   This indicator is measured during a focus group where people are asked directly about the staff approach, using the words 'dignified' and 'caring'.

38   UNICEF Malaria Technical Note 6, February 2003, http://www.unicef.org/health/index_documents.html.

39   Due to the insecticide in the net, those who sleep outside the net but near to it will also be protected against mosquito bites.

40   Bags given to field staff containing essential equipment for survival if forced to flee on foot and stay in the countryside until rescued.

41   Oxfam has a Code of Conduct for all employees – check to see if your agency has one.

42   Adapted from A. Welbourn (1995), South African version.

43   From the Oxfam staff health HIV leaflet.

44   N. Siegfried, M. Muller, J. Volmink, J. Deeks, M. Eggers, N. Low, H. Weiss, S. Walker, P. Williamson (2006) 'Male Circumcision for Prevention of Heterosexual Acquisition of HIV in Men', The Cochrane Database of Systematic Reviews, Issue 3, http://www.cochrane.org/.

Bibliography

General HIV and AIDS resources

Af - AIDS (e-forum), http://www.healthdev.org/eforums/cms/ individual. asp?sid=95&sname=AF-AIDS

Foreman, M. (n.d.) 'ABC of HIV/AIDS' (A glossary of terms), Panos Institute, www.panos.org.

International Centre for Migration and Health (2001) HIV/AIDS and Security, www.icmh.ch

International Clearinghouse on Curriculum for HIV/AIDS Education, www.unesco.org

Murphy, L. L. (2004) 'HIV/AIDS and Humanitarian Action: insights from US Kenya based agencies', London: Overseas Development Institute, www.odi.org.

UNAIDS (2003) 'Population Mobility and AIDS' (Technical Update), February, www.unaids.org.

UNAIDS (2000) 'Voluntary Counselling and Testing' (Technical Update), May, www.unaids.org.

UNAIDS (1997) 'Refugees and AIDS' (Technical Update), September, www.unaids.org.

UNAIDS and WHO (2003) 'AIDS Epidemic Update', December, www.unaids.org/epidemic_update/report_dec01/index.html.

UNHCR (2002) 'HIV/AIDS and Refugees – UNHCR's Strategic Plan 2002–2004', February, www.unhcr.ch.

HIV and emergencies

Holden, S. (2004) *Mainstreaming HIV/AIDS in Development and Humanitarian Programmes*, Oxford: Oxfam.

Holmes, W. (2003) *Protecting the Future: A guide to incorporating HIV prevention, care and support interventions in refugee and post-conflict settings*, International Rescue Committee, and Kumarian Press, www.theirc.org.

IASC (Inter Agency Standing Committee) (2004) 'Guidelines for HIV/AIDS Interventions in Emergency Settings', http://www.who.int/hac/techguidance/pht/hiv/en/index.html.

Smith, A. (2002) 'HIV and emergencies: analysis and recommendations for practice', Humanitarian Practice Network Paper 38, London: Overseas Development Institute.

The Sphere Project (2004) 'Humanitarian Charter and Minimum Standards in Disaster Response', www.sphereproject.org.

UNHCR, WHO, UNAIDS (1995) 'Guidelines for HIV Interventions in Emergency Settings', Geneva, September.

Van Bruaene, M. and A. Doerlemann (2004) 'A Review of DG ECHOs approach to HIV/AIDS', Model Guidelines, ECHO.

Human rights

International Centre for Migration and Health (2000) 'Demobilization and its Implications for HIV/AIDS', October 2000, www.icmh.ch.

UNHCR/UNAIDS (1996) 'HIV/AIDS and Human Rights: International Guidelines', Geneva, September 23–25, www.unaids.org.

Implementation and training

African HIV/AIDS Prevention Initiative (ICA) (2004) 'HIV/AIDS Prevention Education Guide for African Communities: a field guide for lay educators to use in talking with their neighbours about HIV/AIDS', Pact Publications.

Ferron, S., J. Morgan and M. O'Reilly (2002) *Hygiene Promotion: A Practical Manual for Relief and Development*, Rugby: ITDG Publishing.

FHI/PATH (2002) Developing Materials on HIV/AIDS/STIs for Low-Literate Audiences, Washington DC: FHI/PATH.

Fung, V. (ed.) (2004) 'Mapping Made Easy: A guide to understanding and responding to HIV vulnerability', October, UNDP South East Asia HIV and Development Programme.

Gosling, L. and M. Edwards (2002) *Toolkits; A Practical Guide to Assessment, Monitoring, Review, and Evaluation*, London: Save the Children UK.

Rugg, D., G. Peersman, and M. Carael (eds.) (2004) *Global Advances in HIV/AIDS Monitoring and Evaluation*, Jossey-Bass and the American Evaluation Association.

Welbourn, A. (1995) 'Stepping Stones: A training package on HIV/AIDS, gender issues, communication and relationship skills', London: ActionAid, www.actionaid.org/stratshope/ssinfo.html.

Women and gender

Gender - AIDS (e-forum), gender-aids@eforums.healthdev.org.

Oxfam GB (n.d.) 'A Little Gender Handbook for Emergencies or Just Plain Common Sense', (internal document).

UNHCR (1995) 'Sexual Violence Against Refugees: Guidelines on Prevention and Response', Geneva: UNHCR.

UNHCR/UNFPA/WHO (1999) 'Reproductive Health in Refugee Situations: An Inter-agency Field Manual', www.unhcr.ch; www.rhrc.org.

UNICEF (2002) 'HIV/AIDS Education: a Gender Perspective', www.unicef.org.

UNICEF/WHO/USAID (2005) 'HIV and Infant Feeding Counselling Tools: reference guide', Geneva.

WHO (2001) 'Clinical Management of Rape Survivors – A guide to assist in the development of situation-specific protocols', (a draft for field testing, available through the WHO Department of Reproductive Health and Research, www.who.int/reproductive-health).

WHO (2000) 'Reproductive Health During Conflict and Displacement: A guide for programme managers', www.who.int/reproductive-health.

Children, youth, and other vulnerable groups

Mckenna, N. (1996) 'On the margins: men who have sex with men and HIV in the developing world', London: Panos.

UNHCR (2001) 'HIV/AIDS Education for Refugee Youth – The Window of Hope'.

UNICEF (2006) 'Africa's orphaned and vulnerable generations: children affected by AIDS'.

UNICEF (2006) 'Child protection and children affected by AIDS'.

UNICEF (2004) 'Girls, HIV/AIDS and education'.

Food security and nutrition

Emergency Nutrition Network (1999) 'Infant Feeding in Emergencies (Module 1: A manual for emergency relief staff)', ENN, WHO, UNICEF, LINKAGES, IBFAN and others, www.ennonline.net.

FAO (2001) 'The Impact of HIV/AIDS on Food Security', Report to the Committee on World Food Security, 27th session, www.fao.org/docrep/meeting/003/Y0310E.htm.

FAO/WHO (2002) 'Living Well with HIV/AIDS: A manual on nutritional care and support for people living with HIV/AIDS', Rome: FAO.

Fawzi, W. W. et. al. (2004) 'A Randomized Trial of Multivitamin Supplements and HIV Disease Progression and Mortality', *The New England Journal of Medicine* 351(1): 23–32.

UN-ACC Sub-Committee on Nutrition (2001) 'Nutrition and HIV/AIDS', Nutrition Policy Paper No. 20, October, www.acc.unsystem.org/scn/; www.who.int; www.unaids.org.

UNHCR (2004) 'Integration of HIV/AIDS activities with food and nutrition support in refugee settings: specific programme strategies'.

Protection

Slim, H. and Bonwick, A. (2006) *Protection: An ALNAP Guide for Humanitarian Agencies*, Oxford: Oxfam.

Water and sanitation

Kamminga, E. and M.Wegelin-Schuriga, (2003) 'HIV/AIDS and Water, Sanitation and Hygiene: Thematic Overview Paper', Royal Tropical Institute (KIT) and IRC Water and Sanitation Centre, February.

Jones, H. and B. Reed, (2005) *Water and sanitation for disabled people and other vulnerable groups; designing service to improve accessibility*, Loughborough: Water, Engineering and Development Centre (WEDC).

Index

Material in appendices, boxes, and notes is shown as Ap, B, and n after the page numbers

poverty cycle 9
prevention programmes in camps 13
process indicators 48–9
prostitution 70
    in developing countries 15B
protection issues 46B
proxy indicators 22, 48, 104n

'quick run bags' 56

rape
    increased risk in emergencies 16
    increases in cases 10
resource demand, higher for chroni-
    cally ill and carers 13
role models, result of lack of 16

sanitary materials
    important to young girls 16B
    see also menstrual cloths
scoring tool for planners and managers
    24–5, 53
    Aceh example 25B
    used in proposal writing and
        programme planning 24
    which factors increase risk 24
sex for subsistence 15B, 16, 23
    commercial sex workers 15B
    young males 14, 103n
    Zimbabwe example 15B
sex workers, commercial 10, 15B, 70
sexual abuse 16, 25B
    vulnerability of single women and
        child-headed households 36
sexual favours, pressure for in emer-
    gencies 16
sexual intercourse, unprotected, and
    HIV 81Ap
shelter programmes 36
    examples of HIV mainstreaming
        in 36B
Sierra Leone, HIV prevalence, medium
    impact of emergency 12B
small livestock raising 42, 44B
    chicken and egg story 44B

consider risk of avian flu 42, 44B
social factors, increased susceptibility
    to HIV in women and girls 14
Sphere Project 5, 21
    definition of key vulnerable
        groups 13
Sri Lanka, HIV mainstreaming in
    shelter programmes 36B
staff
    induction 51–2, 57–8
    one-day training, objectives 58
stigma/stigmatisation 40, 61
    avoidance of 22, 25–6, 41
    in non-emergency situations 25–6
    of people with HIV and AIDS 17, 18
    recognition of 76–7
STIs 9, 55
substance abuse, in young males 14,
    103n

TBAs, giving appropriate informa-
    tion on HIV transmission 55
traditional herbs 44B
truck drivers 21
    given information and condoms
        for distribution 35B
    risk infection from casual sex 35B
Turkana district, Kenya, programme
    potentially affecting HIV prevalence
    40B

Uganda
    Northern 30B, 36B
    'quick run bags' 56

values clarification, objective 64–5
violence, sexual and gender-based,
    reducing opportunities for 23
voluntary counselling and testing
    centres, require long-term commit-
    ment 54
vulnerability 27
    increased for many by emergencies
        13
    of particular households 26